PRAISE FOR REFLECT

"So you are heading to your fir, murky gel with no visualization of retina and swirls of dark red blood teasing you. Despite the difficult task, you recall the words of your mentor, calming your hands. 'Use the Goldilocks touch,' 'You are the pilot,' and 'You can do this.' Your mind eases and confidently you sail through the case with success.

Ophthalmology is a delicate and precise profession, relying on a strong base of knowledge and sprinkled with tips, pearls, and advice from professors and mentors. Mentors are precious gems that guide you through the 'real world' of ophthalmology on many levels. In this book, Dr. Gupta has brilliantly demonstrated the harmony of understanding basic facts of a patient problem balanced with confidence and experience. Books teach facts, but experience with a trustworthy mentor adds years of confidence. A mentor's advice will dwell in your mind throughout your career, whispering poise as you face challenging cases—'If he can do it, you can too,' 'Improvement begins with I,' and 'Practice makes perfect.'

An honorable salute to Dr. Gupta for realizing and portraying the personal touch of mentoring."

CAROL L. SHIELDS, MD
Ocular Oncology Service, Director, Wills Eye Hospital,
Thomas Jefferson University, Philadelphia, PA

"Rishi has beautifully captured the essence of becoming and being a doctor, from our first days in training to our established practices and surgical lives. He elegantly depicts the memorable *crucial moments* that mold us into doctors outside of the books and protocols. Peppered with quotes that add humor and remarkable insight, this collection of gems will enlighten your view of your patients, mentors, and mentees. For anyone who has been through residency, many of these stories and pearls of wisdom will make you cringe, smile, or outright laugh, sometimes all three! An easy, quick read for anyone, and especially for those entering residency or fellowship—these insights are priceless! This should be required reading for every ophthalmology resident and fellow."

CHARLES C. WYKOFF, MD PHD
Retina Consultants of Houston, Blanton Eye Institute
& Houston Methodist Hospital, Houston, TX

"In his book entitled *Reflections of a Pupil: What Your Med School and Ophthalmology Textbooks Can't Teach You (But What Your Mentors, Colleagues, and Patients Will)*, R. Rishi Gupta summarizes many of his seminal experiences as a resident and fellow and young attending in ophthalmology. The book is elegantly written and the case scenarios are interesting and instructive. Insightful pearls are available on every page and are thoughtfully highlighted by famous quotes and proverbs. The book is thoroughly enjoyable to read and educational at every level. As an academic ophthalmologist already in practice over twenty years, I was able to gain a great deal of insightful information. Congratulations to Rishi on a superb piece of work that will certainly be an important resource for many years to come in the ophthalmology community."

DAVID SARRAF, MD
Clinical Professor of Ophthalmology Retinal Disorders and Ophthalmic Genetics Division Stein Eye Institute, UCLA, Los Angeles, CA

"Dr. Gupta's reflections provide a wonderful balance of practical experiences, words of wisdom, and lessons from positive (and not so positive) moments over the course of his training and early career as an ophthalmologist. Dr. Gupta provides a great balance of inspiration, humility, and words of wisdom. Although this book is most relevant to trainees in the discipline of ophthalmology, his lessons learned and anecdotes will be of value to all healthcare learners, particularly those studying fields involving surgical or medical procedures. The book is well crafted and a very enjoyable read."

DAVID ANDERSON, MD FRCPC
Dean, Faculty of Medicine, Dalhousie University, Halifax, NS

"In this collection of vignettes, Rishi Gupta shares entertaining and educational experiences from his ophthalmologic training. He is certainly leading an examined life, and by relaying his reflections on both the good and the bad along his path, he provides useful insight to all of us, whether we are young ophthalmologists or not. In a book to thank his mentors, Rishi becomes a mentor to us all."

ROBERT L. AVERY, MD
Founder and CEO, California Retina Consultants, Santa Barbara, CA

"Dr. Gupta has captured many of the challenges residents, fellows and new-to-practice physicians face, not only in ophthalmology, but other specialties as well. Drawing on experiences from his own training and early practice, he has succeeded in doing so with humor and easy-to-read prose. His book is encouraging, comes across in a light-hearted way, yet deals with serious issues that will provide much needed support to trainees as they develop the experience and confidence they need to enter practice on their own."

WENDY A. STEWART, MD PHD FRCPC
Paediatric Neurologist, Director of Humanities,
Dalhousie University, Halifax, NS

"This is a wonderful book—it is serious, humorous, insightful, and overall a great read. I believe medical students, residents, colleagues, and team members will all be interested in reading it. As Dr. Gupta demonstrates, every encounter with a patient, learner, and colleague is also an opportunity to learn and grow as a physician and surgeon practicing the art and science of medicine."

JOAN EVANS, PHD
Retired Professor and Director, Communication Skills Program, Faculty of Medicine, Dalhousie University, Halifax, NS

"The greatest book ever written by my son."

RISHI'S MOM

REFLECTIONS OF A PUPIL

R. RISHI GUPTA, MD FRCSC
FOREWORD BY VIVEK R. PATEL, MD

REFLECTIONS OF A PUPIL

What Your Med School and Ophthalmology Textbooks Can't Teach You

(But What Your Mentors, Colleagues, and Patients Will)

OCEAN PLAYGROUND PRESS

AUTHOR'S NOTE

WHILE THE ANECDOTES recounted in this book are based on actual events, conversations, and clinical scenarios, the exact wording of some dialogues was modified for narrative purposes. All named individuals were asked for their permission to allow the author to portray these situations and conversations as they appear. In order to respect and protect the privacy and the identities of patients, identifying details were altered or "composite" patients were created for illustrative purposes.

Copyright © 2018 by R. Rishi Gupta

All rights reserved. No part of this book may be reproduced, stored in a retrieval system or transmitted, in any form or by any means, without the prior written consent of the publisher or a licence from The Canadian Copyright Licensing Agency (Access Copyright). For a copyright licence, visit www.accesscopyright.ca or call toll free to 1-800-893-5777.

ISBN 978-1-99941-970-7 (paperback)
ISBN 978-1-99941-971-4 (ebook)

Some names and identifying details have been changed to protect the privacy of individuals.

This book is not intended as a substitute for the medical advice of physicians. The reader should regularly consult a physician in matters relating to his/her health and particularly with respect to any symptoms that may require diagnosis or medical attention.

Produced by Page Two Books
www.pagetwobooks.com
Cover and interior design by Setareh Ashrafologhalai
Edited by Cynthia N. Lank

rishiguptamd.com/textbooks/

*To Vikram… whatever path you forge in life,
may you always remember to be kind, caring,
and respectful to those around you.*

*In loving memory of
Aditya Vikram Mishra.*

> *"Every teacher is a learner—
> every learner is a teacher."*
>
> UNKNOWN

CONTENTS

Foreword *1*

Preface *3*

1 IN THE OPERATING ROOM AND CLINIC

Never Operate on the Wrong Eye *8*

Make the Jump: From Resident to Fellow *11*

Pick Up the Last Chart *13*

Taking the Leap from Training to Attending *15*

Gotta Have the Goldilocks Touch *18*

Know Your Audience *21*

Put Me In, Coach! *23*

The Only Suture You'll Regret Is the One You Didn't Put In *26*

Don't Smoosh the Eye *28*

We Are the Pilots *30*

There's More Than One Way to Skin a Cat *32*

Embrace Your Inner Detective *34*

He Let 'Em Get Away with It! *36*

Don't Let the Holes Overlap *38*

What If...? *41*

The Active Observer *43*

Don't Take the Report as Gospel *45*

Practice Makes Permanent *49*

The Independent Surgeon *51*

Perfect Is the Enemy of Good *53*

Don't Fight Yourself *55*

Shoot for 100 Percent *57*

Excuse Me for Saying "Oops!" *60*

Last Line of Defense *63*

Don't Get Balderdashed! *65*

Don't Flip-Flop *68*

Provide Anesthesia unto Others as You Would Have It Provided unto Yourself *70*

The Indication for Doing <Blank> Is Having It Cross Your Mind *73*

Bad Form *75*

Keep It Clean *78*

The Only Way to Never Have Surgical Complications Is to Never Operate *81*

Sound Intentions... But Poor Planning and Execution *83*

2 PRACTICE MANAGEMENT AND CAREER PLANNING

Come on Time and Bring Cookies 86
Pick Up the Phone 88
Don't Leave Anyone Out 90
Do a Self-Audit from Time to Time 92
Document Well 94
Who Do You Think You're Dealing With? 96
Minimizing Patient Grievances 98
Privacy Is Dead (and the Internet Killed It!) 101
Extra! Extra! Read All About It! 103
Be Kind to Your Colleagues 105
Let 'Em Know What You Want 107
Don't Just Go with the Flow—Manage It! 110
Fast and Careless Loses the Race 113
Food for Thought 115
The Case That Got Away 117
Don't Be the Dinosaur 120
You Only Find What You Know to Look For 122
Find Efficiencies for Repetitive Tasks 124
Two Thumbs Down 127
Soak in the Business 130
Take Time to Teach 133
What Do *You* Think? 136
Conflicted About Your Interests? 138
Sometimes You Gotta Be the Bad Guy 143

3 PATIENT INTERACTIONS

Be Kind to Your Patients 146

Thank You for Your Patience 149

Web of Lies 151

Walk a Mile in Your Patients' Shoes 153

Keep 'Em Coming Back 155

Great Expectations 158

Get Your Head Out of That Screen! 160

Don't Get Too Cozy 162

Truly Informed Decisions 165

Make the Connection 169

Always Validate Your Patient's Experience 172

Can You Say That Again, But This Time So It Makes Sense? 174

That Made Sense! But Now I Don't Remember Any of It... 176

I Gotta Feeling 178

Tough Question! 180

Better Than the Boss 183

What's the (Full) Story, Morning Glory? 185

You Can Choose Your Friends, But You Can't Choose Your Patients 188

You Can't Win 'Em All 190

Worst Behavior 192

4 LIFE LESSONS

"A Goal Without a Plan Is a Wish" *196*

Make Your Slope a Little Steeper *198*

What's Your Greatest Strength? *200*

If We Were All the Same,
It'd Be a Boring World *202*

Sometimes the Squeaky Wheel Gets
the Grease, and Sometimes It Gets Replaced *205*

Go Where You Want to Be *208*

Please, Tell Me How You *Really* Feel *210*

Time Flies (Make Sure You're On Board) *213*

If He Can Do It, I Can Too! *216*

Always Look Like a Winner *218*

Learn to Say No *220*

These Are My Confessions *223*

I Did Everything I Could *226*

Don't Forget! *228*

Don't Let the Fall Crush You *230*

An Error Is Wasted If You Don't
Learn from It *232*

No Regrets *235*

How Do You Deal with Defeat? *237*

Don't Live in Relative Poverty *239*

Attend Your Own Funeral *241*

Reflections of a Pupil *243*

Acknowledgments *245*

FOREWORD

WE ALL HAD a vision of what it would be like to be a doctor. Some of us started dreaming in childhood, others saw it first through the eyes of a physician parent, and a few just stumbled across it when already entrenched in another career. Regardless of how we got here, or in what stage in our careers we may be, I think we can all agree that the practice of medicine is simultaneously humbling yet empowering, technical yet artistic, and full of lessons each and every day.

Although we each carry with us personal lessons learned over the years, in my mind, Dr. Gupta is the perfect person to write this book. I first met Rishi when I became one of his newest attendings during his early years as an ophthalmology resident at the University of Ottawa. His talents as a student and physician were obvious, but what shone through just as brightly was his innate ability to see the bigger picture. Experiences only become insights if they are understood; Rishi uncovers the message hidden in each encounter—positive or negative, serious or casual—and has the ability to tap into the deeper lesson. This compilation of anecdotes and experiences cuts to the heart of what it means to be a physician.

By now, you have read countless articles, textbooks, and original scientific works, and you will continue to consume medical literature at a torrid pace over the course of your career. But, you will rarely come across a source like this, which allows you to step away from the specific subject matter for a moment, yet still be as relevant and important to your career in medicine as anything you may read in your chosen field.

If you're just beginning your path as a physician, you'll be grateful for these pearls of wisdom, and recall them with familiarity and comfort when such a scenario inevitably arrives. If you're in the middle of your career, like I am, I can tell you each excerpt is absolutely germane to the everyday practice of medicine and a great reminder of lessons we *should* have learned along the way. And for the seasoned clinician in the twilight of one's career, I can only suspect that Dr. Gupta's *Reflections of a Pupil* reads much like an anthology of your own career, as you look back on all that the privilege of being a physician has taught you.

VIVEK R. PATEL, MD
Associate Professor
Director, Neuro-ophthalmology and Adult Strabismus
Residency Program Director
USC Roski Eye Institute, Keck School of Medicine
University of Southern California
Los Angeles, California

PREFACE

OPHTHALMOLOGY RESIDENTS, FELLOWS, and junior attendings have ready access to a wealth of textbooks dedicated to helping expand the technical aspects of their medical and surgical knowledge. But no textbook or article can capture those clinical pearls and life lessons that are imparted to us by our teachers, mentors, and patients. Yet these are as essential to us becoming caring, safe, conscientious, and efficient surgeons as the technical skills we learn and hone over so many years of training.

This book is a tapestry of lessons that I have learned on my own journey through the art and science of medicine. It is my hope that this collection will provide food for thought for the junior physician who, through training, has been armed with all the medical knowledge and technical aspects for a successful practice, but perhaps may still benefit from self-reflection in order to grow to his or her full potential. My advice is not intended to be prescriptive but simply thought provoking, as there is always more than one way to approach a given situation.

Most people in the apprenticeship model of medicine can recall critical heart-to-heart conversations—often right after the difficult case, the missed diagnosis, or the less-than-ideal patient interaction. Often the junior physician in these scenarios is in a vulnerable place. During these crucial moments, a capable and compassionate mentor can have a very positive and lasting influence. If we are lucky, we will cross paths with these great mentors during our training: they are very supportive; they recognize that when things don't evolve in an ideal manner, it's all part of the process of growing as a clinician and surgeon; and they help us focus on how things could have been handled differently, so that we have a chance to do better the next time. I hope the anecdotes in this book resemble the positive conversations about tough topics that occur between such mentors and their colleagues and students in the hallways of hospitals around the world.

While the chapters are loosely organized around the themes of the operating room and clinic, practice management and career planning, patient interactions, and life lessons, our daily lives and medical practice aren't organized in these neat categories. So please read this book from front to back, or back to front, or randomly through whichever titles or passages catch your eye first. I hope you can consume it in small bites as your busy life allows. This is a "something for everyone" offering. As such, not every passage will necessarily resonate with you, depending on your specialty, practice profile, and stage of career. However, I am confident that you will come across at least one chapter that will make you think about approaching patient care, mentoring, or education in a different way. And don't worry if you can't define (or pronounce) "phacoemulsification" or "rhegmatogenous"—that's not the focus of the lessons (and Dr. Google is just a click away if you're curious!).

I hope that as you move from junior attending to seasoned senior ophthalmologist, you will be generous to those junior to you and that you will take the time to teach and mentor. Your interactions will have a significant impact on them, just as those with whom you trained influenced you. Each encounter with a patient or a colleague is a chance for you to learn and grow, a chance to showcase not only your clinical acumen and surgical expertise but your personal qualities—empathy, compassion, honesty, kindness, and humility. I also hope you will strive for that elusive work-life balance. Don't allow yourself to be pulled in so many directions that you are actually pulled apart. Yes, your patients need you, but your family and friends do too.

Finally, it is inevitable that, one day, you will be sitting in the patient's chair. Strive to be the type of doctor you want to be sitting across from when that day comes.

R. RISHI GUPTA
Halifax, Nova Scotia

1

IN THE OPERATING ROOM AND CLINIC

"Fortune favors the prepared mind."
LOUIS PASTEUR

NEVER OPERATE
ON THE WRONG EYE

I GAZED AROUND the room at the other first-year surgical retina fellows sitting in the auditorium. It was August 2011 and we were at the Massachusetts Eye and Ear Infirmary for the first annual Fellow's Vitrectomy course. Dr. Donald D'Amico, chairman of ophthalmology at Weill Cornell Medical College, made his way to the podium. I do not remember all the details about his talk now, but I do remember his first sentence. While somehow simultaneously staring directly into each of our eyes, he soberly stated, "Never operate on the wrong eye. There are very few ways to get kicked out of fellowship, but that is one of them." That moment left a deep impression on me. I must have repeated that phrase to myself before starting every case for about a year.

My fellowship director, Dr. Michael Kapusta—not known for being shy with his words—reinforced this concept. "Nothing about this should be casual," he said firmly to me on one of my first days. "Don't just look at the list for the operating room—what if someone entered it wrong? You need to check the name, the date of birth, the medical record number, the patient's wristband, your note on the chart, the referring doctor's note, *and* the list on the wall. Double-check and then triple-check! And you do it yourself—don't take the word of the resident or the nurse and, in a hurry, block the wrong eye. In this operating room, the onus is on you to make sure everything goes right."

Very early in my fellowship I was operating on a patient with diabetes for a dense nonclearing vitreous hemorrhage. He had had a previous vitrectomy one year before. After confirming proper positioning of the infusion line and opening it, I placed the second trocar. At the time, we were using nonvalved ports so fluid gushed from the port. I didn't think anything of it and soon after plugging that port, I placed my last trocar. When I pulled in the BIOM lens, my heart stopped. There was very little vitreous hemorrhage! Was I in the wrong eye?! Had I just done what Dr. D'Amico told me not to do? I saw my whole career disappearing before my eyes. But wait, before starting the case, hadn't I checked the eye, the patient, and the chart? I pulled away from the oculars of the microscope and gazed down at the drapes. Yes, this was the correct eye. I got out of my seat and confirmed it against the chart again. Suddenly it dawned on me that most of the hemorrhage had essentially washed out of the eye once all the ports were in place, as is typical in a previously vitrectomized eye. Phew! I removed residual vitreous with scleral depression, added some additional laser, and closed up.

Almost all operating rooms now have multiple checks to ensure that the correct side is being prepared for the operation. Dr. Kapusta's point is an important one, however. This system is only as good as the first point of entry. Say your surgical booking staff erroneously enters that you are supposed to do surgery on Mr. H.'s right eye, when it is actually his left eye. Unless you catch that error, there is an amazing mechanism in place to set you up for failure. Everyone in the preoperative area will check and double-check the list and prepare

Mr. H.'s incorrect eye. The nurses in the operating room will go by the list and plan for the eye that was booked. The only two people at this point who can save you (and Mr. H.'s good eye) are you and Mr. H. himself. Not infrequently, however, Mr. H. may not be able to help you, as he is either too anxious, too scared, or (as with many of our elderly patients) too forgetful to remember which eye is supposed to be done.

So in addition to checking with the patient, always double-check against other information available. Make sure the referring doctor's note, your note, and the OR list that your surgical coordinator created all align. If you have a preoperative image such as an OCT or color photograph that you can use to verify the correct eye, all the better.

Be diligent and never operate on the wrong eye!

MAKE THE JUMP: FROM RESIDENT TO FELLOW

DURING RESIDENCY, YOU have four short years to learn, operate, and hone your skills (although sometimes it feels like it's not going fast enough!). However, your fellowship's even more contracted timeline means that time will fly by quickly. You will have a finite amount of time to become as comfortable, knowledgeable, and experienced as possible before you will be out on your own and considered the expert subspecialist. Make sure that you are ready from day one to dive in!

It can be a tough transition from being a senior resident, comfortable in your shoes, to being the new person in an unfamiliar environment, learning new skills. In your early surgical rotations in residency, you dealt with the frustrations of perfecting your capsulorhexis and learning to chop, and by the end, you felt comfortable with cataract surgery. Get ready to start from the bottom again! If you've moved to a new institution to train, all the goodwill you built up over residency disappears; you are starting with a clean slate again. You have to prove once more that you are conscientious, hard-working, efficient, and dependable.

Prior to your start date, try to connect with the current fellows. Pick their brains about how best to prepare, the various staff members' expectations, how to get the most out of the experience, and what they would have done differently. Many programs will encourage you to be involved in research. Ask the previous fellows if there are any specific supervisors and projects they would recommend. Unless you are organized from day one, time will slip away.

Your fellowship can be one of the most daunting and stressful times of your career. You will be challenged surgically, intellectually, and emotionally. We put a significant amount of pressure on ourselves to excel and do well. While we want to make sure the patient has an optimal outcome, we also know that there is a finite time for us to learn and gain the experience to allow us to be confident and comfortable once we are out on our own. Know your limits and slowly work to improve upon them.

During residency, you were likely one of a relatively large group. As the number of fellows is much smaller, you cannot hide! In fact, you may be the only one and, practically speaking and quite possibly, be responsible for running the service. In the same way that you likely looked to the fellow for guidance when you were a resident, the residents will be looking to you. Work hard. Be known for picking up the last chart in clinic and not just leaving it for someone else. Dress and carry yourself in a professional manner. Pay close attention to how your mentors communicate with their patients. Note how they package information on diagnosis, prognosis, and risks and benefits of treatments and how they convey this to patients. Take the best of the group and formulate your own approach going forward.

My best piece of advice for your fellowship—jump in with both feet and carpe diem!

PICK UP
THE LAST CHART

"All right, let's see what's left," I said to myself. I checked the charts of the patients who were still waiting to be seen.

"Hmm... new-onset vaginal bleed... ooooor... bright red blood per rectum... Fantastic," I said with a deep sigh.

Being an ophthalmology resident in the emergency room during one's rotating internship year can sometimes be... well... uncomfortable. In fact, truth be told, one of the main reasons I applied to ophthalmology was so I would not have to work up patients with vaginal or rectal bleeding!

"Maybe I should lock myself in the bathroom until my shift is over?" I asked myself. In my mind, I heard the voice of a mentor of mine. "Pick up the last chart," he always used to say. "OK, OK, OK," I said out loud. "Rectal bleed it is!"

One day in the clinic, a few of us overheard a resident who was presenting to an attending say that the patient had "short-gut syndrome." The resident next to me murmured, "Did he say short-cut syndrome? Because I know someone who has that." I was surprised that I immediately knew to whom he was referring—this individual was known for always finding a way out of doing things.

When working in a group setting with multiple residents, fellows, and attendings, there is sometimes the tendency to drag one's feet, knowing that eventually the tasks will get done by someone else in the team. Fight this feeling! If everyone makes a habit of picking up the last chart and working hard, everything will move much more efficiently.

Don't allow your actions to make people think that you are not hard-working. Always go the extra mile!

TAKING THE LEAP FROM TRAINING TO ATTENDING

AFTER YEARS OF hard work, the day finally arrives—your training is over and you are now an attending! The shift from the end of your fellowship (or residency) to the beginning of independent practice brings with it one substantial change: the responsibility now becomes *all* yours. The safety net is gone. No more leaving the final decision to someone else. No more reminders from your attending that it is always important with a patient presenting with X to do a, b, and c. Now if you see a patient with an iatrogenic complication, a complicated pathology, or a difficult personality, they will stay with you. You are no longer rotating to another site or service—it's all you now!

Early in your last year of training, regularly ask yourself, "What would I do next if I were out on my own?" When someone else is there to guide us or correct us, too often our minds get lazy and we go into autopilot. Not infrequently, we allow the person looking over our shoulder to remind us of details that we should have thought of. When you have someone to lean on who has more responsibility, it's easy to say, "Oh yeah…" when they prompt you to do something. But when you're on your own, if you don't think of it, it won't happen! While you still have your supervisors, push yourself to be better prepared for being out in the jungle on your own.

As a newly minted attending, nowhere will you feel the weight of responsibility more than in the operating room. In clinic, if a case is complicated, you always have the time to think more, to bring the patient back in for a follow-up, or to order more tests or imaging. The operating room functions very differently and demands an immediacy and definitiveness to your decisions, or else the day will not progress and cases will get canceled. During your training, if you were unable to surgically accomplish something in a safe manner, you and the attending could switch seats. This luxury, of course, disappears when *you* are the attending. The operating room is a very lonely place when you struggle with a difficult case and there is no one more senior to whom you can hand over the reins. It can be all the more nerve-wracking when a resident or medical student is watching and asking you questions. Get used to this concept becoming a reality very quickly.

If you accept a position in a hospital in which you have not operated before, do not be surprised if your first day in the operating room feels somewhat awkward. Working in a new space with new nurses and possibly different instruments, equipment, and microscope will take some getting used to. It brings a whole new meaning to the saying "There's no place like home."

Budget for this and make sure your first day in the new environment is lightly booked with straightforward cases. The first time you have a complication while on your own, your heart will likely be pounding, and you will feel like the walls are caving in on you. Take a deep breath. Remember that you have been well trained and that you can handle this. Calm your mind and work through it step by step. It is not uncommon to second-guess decisions that just a few months prior as a fellow, you would not have thought twice about. Before leaving the patient interaction or operating room, take a second to ask yourself, "Have I forgotten anything?"

In addition, you will probably encounter things in independent practice that you did not experience during your training. Be prepared to think on your feet. Your training gave you the skills to be able to manage things on your own. And if ever you are really stuck, just think "What would _____ do?" and insert your smartest attending's initials in the space!

GOTTA HAVE
THE GOLDILOCKS TOUCH

THE EYE IS a delicate organ. Ophthalmic surgery demands a high level of dexterity and subtlety of movement in order to achieve consistent and high-quality outcomes. Microns often make the difference between success and complications. Make the corneal wound too short in cataract surgery and now you are dealing with iris prolapse. Step a little too aggressively on the pedal during phacoemulsification and suddenly you are managing vitreous loss.

Somehow, through your training and early years of independent practice, you have to find that fine balance between being too timid and too aggressive. It takes a significant amount of time to learn how much tension and force the tissues can handle. What is appropriate in one case may not be advisable in another case due to variations in patient anatomy. Be conscious of this as you are operating and when watching others operate live or on video, and continue to refine your approach.

During residency and fellowship, you are constantly assessed and your surgical skills are always under the microscope (literally!). For a multitude of reasons, it is not always easy for an attending to sit at the sidescope and watch you operate. If you are overly aggressive, they will be even less keen to stay at the assistant's scope. At the same time, you can't be so timid that the surgery fails to move forward at a reasonable pace. Find the balance and you will be rewarded with more opportunities to grow.

I can still remember the first time I made a corneal incision for cataract surgery on a live patient. My heart was pounding. My own corneas were drying out because I could not blink due to the intensity of the situation. Not knowing the feel of the tissue, I was so gentle. For the attending looking on, it probably felt like an eternity for the blade to actually enter the eye. With each case after that, however, I made a point of internalizing the feel of the movement and force required, in order to become more efficient without being overly aggressive.

By the end of residency, a corneal incision (and cataract surgery) was second nature. Then I got to start the process all over again with fellowship! When I switched chairs to do my first internal limiting membrane (ILM) peel for a macular hole, I could not even touch the surface of the retina! My forceps would come close and then my brain would tell my hand to stop and close the forceps, and I'd grab nothing! It was like there was a force field protecting the ILM and preventing me from coming closer; I was so scared of doing something wrong.

Often the first try in the operating room may not feel like a success. However, if you do not create a problem, look at it as a relative success. Each experience gives you more information about the approach and how to hold the instruments, focus the microscope, and achieve the appropriate magnification. At first, always err on the side of being too gentle. As you get to do more cases, push yourself to be more assertive with your movements. If you end up being too aggressive, dial things back. Eventually you'll find yourself in the sweet spot where you have the Goldilocks touch! Not too timid, not too aggressive, but juuuuust right!

KNOW YOUR AUDIENCE

NO ONE LIKES to give up control, so watching another person operate on your patient can be tough! As a fellow or resident, the best way for you to allow your attending to feel in control while at the assistant scope is to perform the steps exactly as he or she would. Do things in the same order. Use the same instruments. Try to match the pace of their movements inside and around the eye. Employ the same direction and magnitude of force. Your goal should be to try to make each step of the surgery look exactly as it would if your attending were doing the procedure, such that a masked observer would not be able to tell the difference. What's most important, however, is to respond without delay to your attendings' guidance while they watch you operate. If they say "stop" but you want to push just a little further, *stop*. Even if you have to switch chairs, don't worry: you'll get another chance. For attendings at the sidescope, there is nothing more disconcerting than feeling that the person they're guiding is not responding quickly to their directions. Attendings who feel a loss of control may be hesitant to hand over the reins next time.

Take detailed notes about exactly how each of your attendings likes to approach every stage of surgery. You may be surprised at how different they can be. In fact, you may see two of your attendings tackle a specific step in a completely opposite way! When I was in residency training, one of my cataract mentors insisted on only minimal rotation of the nucleus after hydrodissection, as he believed that this movement caused the greatest stress on the zonules. Another one of my attendings encouraged the opposite and would rotate the nucleus vigorously. To stay in the surgeon's chair, I had to know my audience and operate accordingly. Understanding *why* a surgeon performs steps a certain way will help you select the approach that makes the most sense in your mind when you are an attending. Surgeons are very anecdotal beings. Many of the tips you receive over your training likely relate directly to a complication that arose when they did things differently and what they learned from the experience. Pay attention and you can benefit greatly from these tips!

After your training, you will be all on your own for the rest of your career. You'll have tons of time then to stay in the main chair. In fact, there will be times when you probably won't want to be there and will wish for a switch! You only have a finite time with your attendings, so be smart and make the most of it.

PUT ME IN, COACH!

I WAS PARTWAY through my residency and becoming more comfortable with each step of cataract surgery. My main surgery rotation had just started and I was excited to continue improving my skills and increasing my experience. As it was my first time working with this particular attending, I watched the first few surgeries. He had identified a case later in the morning that he felt was at an appropriate level for me. Happily, the patient consented for me to perform the operation, and everything went great! That is, until we tested the incision at the end of the case. The wound I had crafted was a little short and, as a result, was not self-sealing. While all the cataract surgeries that I had observed or participated in up to this point had been sutureless, here was an instance where a stitch would be needed to close the wound and reduce the risk of infection.

"Throw in a suture," said my attending.

The great scientist Louis Pasteur said that "fortune favors the prepared mind." My mind was unfortunately not prepared to suture the cornea! I'd never had to do it with any of my other cases. Since this scenario was so uncommon, I hadn't spent much time focusing on corneal sutures in the wet lab, and I was now realizing that I should have.

Now, for those of you who have never closed a corneal wound, the first thing I will tell you is that the suture we use is *tiny*. It is thinner than a human hair! In fact, unless you join us at the microscope to watch our work, from a distance it might look like we aren't doing anything at all. Due to the delicate nature of the fine thread, it is not uncommon to break a suture or two as we learn what degree of tension these fragile fibers can withstand. And now imagine that as you carefully try to guide this wisp of material into a knot without snapping it, the tiny needle to which it is attached becomes magnetized and therefore defiant to actually being grasped by the needle driver. This happens routinely. In fact, it can comically look like the needle has come alive; every time the surgeon tries to grab the needle, it jumps out of the way.

OK. You can do this. Deep breath. I passed the needle through both sides of the incision. So far so good. Next I slowly pulled the suture through, hoping to leave a few millimeters so that it would be easier to tie the knot. *Darn!* I managed to pull the thread all the way through! *OK, start over. You can do this.* I passed the needle through both sides of the incision. *Perfect.* I left ample suture on the far side of the incision. Next I looped the suture three times around my tying forceps. *OK, brain, don't burn out here. We need to keep these loops on the forceps and slowly move toward the free end of the suture. OK, we're in good position. Now we need to open the teeth of the forceps just slightly and grab that free end.* The forceps opened too wide. *No! No! No!* I helplessly watched the suture pull all the way through the cornea again. Agony. I was now acutely aware of the clock ticking in the room and felt the eyes of everyone in the OR staring at me. As I fumbled to grab the needle to start all over again, at the last second it would jump away.

My attending decided to put me out of my (and his) misery. "Why don't we switch chairs?"

After the patient was brought back to the postoperative recovery room, my attending and I found a quiet area and he said to me, "Do you watch football?"

"Yes," I replied.

"You know who has the hardest job? The guy coming off the bench to replace the injured quarterback. He's not warmed up, he hasn't had any reps during a game that mattered in months, and yet, if he's good, he's ready. He says, 'Put me in, Coach!' Being a surgeon-in-training is sort of like being a back-up quarterback. You never know when you're going to have the chance to jump in and play."

Message received. You can't succeed if you only know half the playbook. Just like the quarterback coming off the bench, we've got to be prepared for every opportunity.

THE ONLY SUTURE YOU'LL REGRET IS THE ONE YOU DIDN'T PUT IN

IN THE PAST decades, cataract surgery and retina surgery have undergone significant technological evolutions that have allowed for efficient surgery through smaller and smaller wounds. Sutureless small-incision surgery is now commonplace. As a result, today's trainees do not gain the same level of comfort, speed, and confidence in their suturing skills as their predecessors did. While sutureless wounds save time, they can, in a small minority of cases, lead to severe complications.

This was a lesson I learned firsthand during my fellowship training. We operated without issue on a patient for a macular hole. At the end of surgery, his wounds had appeared to be self-sealing and therefore were not sutured. However, by the postoperative day one visit, he had developed a massive suprachoroidal hemorrhage in the operated eye. He'd evidently had some leakage through the wounds and resultant hypotony, and he'd suffered this devastating bleed in turn. I felt terrible about this rare occurrence and wished that we had sutured all of his sclerotomies. I could not help but wonder if doing so would have prevented this uncommon event from occurring in this highly myopic patient. Fortunately, once the hemorrhage settled down, he had a very favorable outcome.

Hypotony and wound leaks are the enemy! If you worry that your patient will ignore instructions and rub their eye after cataract surgery, secure the wound at the end of the case. It's better to do this than to find yourself staring at iris hanging out of the wound on postoperative day one! If your patient is at risk for suprachoroidal hemorrhage, consider suturing. If your patient is monocular, consider sewing up the incision. If you ever have any doubts, take the extra minute and put in a suture. The only suture you'll regret is the one that you didn't put in!

DON'T SMOOSH
THE EYE

"SEE HOW YOU'RE about to smoosh the eye? Please don't smoosh the eye..." I was teaching one of our residents how to suture the conjunctiva closed after a scleral buckle. As he focused intently on the needle driver in his right hand, the forceps in his wandering left hand were about to put pressure on the cornea. I passed on wisdom that I received early in my residency when my chopper would drift during cataract surgery: "Always be aware of what your other hand is doing when it is outside of your immediate attention." The resident could not have given a more honest and insightful response: "I know that's simple, but it sure as hell ain't easy."

Learning ophthalmic surgery is a demanding undertaking. There are not many other specialties in which a surgeon commonly employs all four limbs when operating! Getting accustomed to using one foot to control the microscope, one foot for phacoemulsification, and two hands to disassemble a nucleus in a very small space is quite a feat when you step back and think about it.

It is easy to become so engrossed with one area of the surgical field that we do not notice what is happening in another.

When we are concentrating, we risk developing tunnel vision—like a horse wearing blinders. This is particularly true when we are doing something new or difficult. A drifting instrument can cause complications. Delayed recognition of matters such as bleeding or anterior chamber shallowing can lead to a more involved and challenging case.

After becoming used to cataract surgery through residency, I had to remind myself of this lesson all over again while learning retina surgery during fellowship. In the initial stages of this training, ensuring that my left hand was properly lighting the macula so that my right hand could accomplish an ILM peel was a whole new mental exercise. So was performing bimanual surgery for a diabetic tractional retinal detachment.

We should challenge ourselves to always be aware of what is happening not just in the full surgical field of the microscope but throughout the operating room as a whole. We have to be alert to identify if our instruments are defective or improperly set up, or if the machines sound abnormal or respond inappropriately. We need to be able to recognize if the patient is feeling uncomfortable and is about to move. We must have a good sense of the interpersonal dynamics in the room: Who is working with us? Will there be any challenges as a result? For example, will a medical student be observing or will you be working with a new nurse for the first time?

Being aware will make us better surgeons for our patients. This skill develops with practice but only if we're committed to being on highest alert to everything that is going on around us.

WE ARE THE PILOTS

IN THE OPERATING room, the responsibility for our patients' outcomes lands squarely on our shoulders. The other team members—nurses, anesthetists, technicians, cleaners, porters—all perform their respective vital roles. However, at the end of the day, we are accountable for safeguarding our patients' eyes and making sure that everything goes OK. It is up to us to ensure that, from takeoff to landing, every step proceeds toward the best possible outcome. If issues arise, our job, as the pilots, is to manage the situation and calmly guide those around us.

Many distractions and unexpected obstacles can threaten our attention to the task at hand. There may be medical students, residents, or industry representatives joining us and asking questions that divert our attention. Inexperienced nurses or nurses-in-training may not be completely familiar with the instruments and set-up, and they may not respond as swiftly as we need or expect. Potentially even more hazardous, connections may not be properly tightened or correctly attached. Have you ever been passed an instrument that is damaged and performs suboptimally or been told that a disposable is unavailable and back-ordered? We need to be nimble enough to react to these unanticipated situations and to compensate for them.

At times, we may struggle with the patients themselves—either due to a difficult personality or as a result of their disinhibitions after being sedated. Any surgeon who has done enough cases under local anesthesia knows all too well the dangers of a patient being *too* sedated or not sedated *enough*. Complicating our mission is the patient's anatomy itself, which may be abnormal and render the case more challenging.

Finally, we are often fighting ourselves. Perhaps things are stressful at home and we haven't gotten enough sleep. Maybe we are frustrated with a colleague's behavior and this is playing on our minds. It could be that we are catching a flight at the end of the day for an exciting vacation and our thoughts are already on the beach. The onus is on us to calm our minds and to compartmentalize our stress, worries, and daydreams in order to focus on the task at hand. Through all of these potential obstacles, our duty is to try to achieve the outcome the patient deserves.

Be polite with the team when conveying what you need to perform the operation safely. Everyone wants what is best for the patient. If you make your requests in a nice way, and explain the benefits for the patient, everyone will be understanding. If you need quiet, ask for silence "please." If you need the room to be dark in order to improve your visualization, ask someone to please turn off the lights. Do whatever you feel you need to do to accomplish the task.

At the end of the day, the onus is on you to deal with any issues and safely land the plane.

THERE'S MORE THAN ONE WAY TO SKIN A CAT

FIRST OF ALL, why on earth you'd want to skin a cat is beyond me. That said, I guess it's good to know that there are multiple ways of doing so.

Versatility is a valuable skill, both in the clinic and the operating room. Versatility is cultivated by seeking out different styles and tactics—by working with your various mentors, attending conferences, and watching videos. Expose yourself to diverse approaches, and, over time, you can mesh together what works best in your hands with your environment, resources, and patient population.

During my vitreoretinal fellowship training, I would regularly scleral depress for my attending (and vice versa) to allow for a very thorough shave of the vitreous base. When I started as an attending at a new hospital, I quickly realized that there was no one available who was trained to perform this role while I operated. I consulted colleagues and researched strategies to scleral depress solo. I was amazed at how many different ways had been thought of and described. Necessity is indeed the mother of invention! I tested out a few approaches and settled on the one that felt best in my hands.

If you are stuck in your ways and a new situation comes up, you will have a hard time adapting and feeling comfortable. One of my mentors told me that each year he traveled to a different city and joined a fellow ophthalmologist in their clinic and operating room. What a great idea! Not only do you get to spend time with a colleague and pick their brain about how they would manage various complicated scenarios, but you can also see up close and personal how they run their clinic and OR. You stand to learn not just about the medical and surgical sides of a practice but also about the practice management and teaching sides (and likely a few general life lessons as well). I started doing this and decided to join colleagues in my own subspecialty of medical and surgical retina, as well as to branch out and join other subspecialists in ophthalmology. I spent some time with a few colleagues who perform complex anterior segment work to see how their perspectives could complement my practice. I challenge you to walk away from such experiences without picking up at least one interesting tip that you want to try in your own practice!

By the time I had finished my first year of independent practice, I had performed surgery in eight different operating rooms in multiple cities (including sites where I had done training). Each OR felt foreign the first time I operated in it. No two ORs had the exact same physical layout, stretchers, lighting, machines, instruments, microscope, or (of course) nurses and anesthesiologists. While it is always nice to have that "home-field advantage" feeling, if you invest in versatility, you'll be better poised to adapt to change when you need to.

EMBRACE YOUR INNER DETECTIVE

WE CAN ESSENTIALLY break down the consults that we receive into two basic categories. We've got the "I know what this is, but since you've got the expertise, can you please treat it?" and then there's the "What the heck caused this and should I be worried about it??"

Many of these referrals to ophthalmology are "spot diagnoses." One look at the pathology is often all the experienced practitioner needs to clinch the diagnosis. Peering through the clear window provided by the cornea, we can observe single white blood cells floating around the anterior chamber in times of inflammation. Focus a little deeper into the eye with a lens, and in instances of retinal artery occlusion, we can sometimes discern individual red blood cells marching in single file. Some of the coolest aspects of the specialty are its visual nature and captivating microscopic details. (Even after years of being in ophthalmology, these things still amaze me when I stop to think about them.)

However, expert pattern recognition has its limits, as the eye has only so many ways of responding to the variety of possible insults. Certain presentations, therefore, may look the same (especially in their late stages) and can be challenging to diagnose. "What the heck happened here and should

I be worried??" consults usually require additional brain power and detective work. We need to analyze for clues, complement these with the patient's (hopefully somewhat accurate) clinical history, and try to come up with a determination of the etiology. If we are lucky, there might be previous documentation or photographs to guide us with respect to the lesion's evolution over time.

Usually, patients present to their doctor early or midway through the course of their disease. At times, however, they present late because they were either asymptomatic and unaware of the issue or, in some cases, not interested or worried enough to seek medical care. Sometimes we are consulted to examine the equivalent of a generic scar. Now, a lot of things can cause a scar: trauma, inflammation, infection, or an ischemic event, to name a few. In the active stage of disease or soon after trauma, clinical signs and diagnostic tests often help us determine the cause. But when we're left with only a scar to work with, it can be more challenging to work backward and determine the cause. For example, in a patient with optic disc edema and macular star, there is a high probability of a diagnosis of neuroretinitis secondary to *Bartonella*. However, if the same patient were to present much later, with only optic disc pallor once the healing response had occurred, a much broader differential and more detective work would be needed to explain what had happened.

So, while most of your consults may be straightforward, some cases will demand more detective work. As you try to reverse engineer what caused this patient's legacy of disease, consider all possibilities and maintain a wide differential. Do your best Sherlock Holmes impression and hope that the diagnosis becomes "elementary." It's no coincidence that the great author Sir Arthur Conan Doyle pursued ophthalmology at one point!

HE LET 'EM GET AWAY WITH IT!

AFTER SURGERY, MOST people want to return to their regular life as soon as possible. We would too! It's a bummer being laid up and being asked to stay still and quiet while things heal. In their quest to get back to work, hobbies, and day-to-day life, some patients may bargain with you or even seek your blessings for the craziest things. We need to anticipate this and do our best to prevent them from (unintentionally) undoing their own surgery or medical treatment. "Come on, doc!" one guy said to me in the OR right after I finished his surgery for a macular hole. "No," I replied. "You cannot go play hockey with the boys tonight!"

When we meet with patients after surgery, they have their list of questions that typically starts with "When can I start doing ___ again?" (I give every patient a postoperative educational sheet that covers most of these questions, and I am always interested in how many new questions come up.) There are generally two types of approaches taken by surgeons with respect to postop directions—conservative or relaxed. Often these directions mirror the physician's personality. There are cataract surgeons who still place restrictions on patients with regard to not bending their head down or lifting anything more than ten pounds. There are others who tell their patients they can be on the golf course the next day. Some retina surgeons instruct their patients to keep strict face-down positioning for one to two weeks after macular hole surgery, while others find that to be overkill.

During my residency, I worked with a corneal surgeon whose approach and words always stuck with me. Dr. Kashif Baig, then assistant professor at the University of Ottawa Eye Institute, would tell his patients, "Don't think, 'What can I get away with?' Change your mindset and think, 'What can I do to maximize the chances that this heals well and to minimize the chances that I develop any problems or complications?'" Most surgeons who have done enough cases don't indulge patients' "What can I get away with?" mentality.

Make sure that your patients understand that surgery is serious business. Don't let them undo your fine work by being too lax with them!

DON'T LET THE HOLES OVERLAP

THE "SWISS CHEESE model" of accident causation[1] is regularly discussed in quality-improvement literature. Essentially, each slice of cheese is a layer of protection from the occurrence of an adverse event, with the holes in the cheese representing vulnerabilities. While any single error may not result in failure, multiple faults sequentially lining up will doom the process.

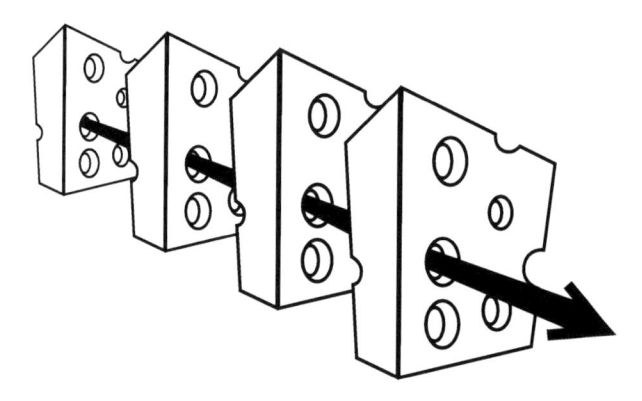

---

[1] J. Reason, "Human Error: Models and Management," *BMJ* no. 320 (2000): 768–770.

A surgeon I met at a conference recounted a story to me that illustrates this model well. Several unfortunate circumstances led to an intraocular lens (IOL) with an incorrect power being implanted into a patient's eye during cataract surgery. The technician who did the eye measurements was new, with only a modest amount of experience, and working alone for the first time. The machine being used by this novice technician had been recently purchased and was relatively unfamiliar to the whole group. Unfortunately, a large standard deviation in the patient's axial length measurement was not recognized or highlighted by the technician, nor was it identified by the surgeon, who was unacquainted with the new machine's printout. An emergency on-call phone consult distracted the surgeon immediately prior to the case. As a result, when the senior resident in the operating room picked the IOL, the attending neglected to double-check it. In retrospect, the IOL did not make sense in light of the patient's refraction or when compared to his other eye's measurements. So... a new unsupervised technician, an unfamiliar printout, an eager resident, and a surgeon whose attention was being pulled away for an emergency culminated in a fixable but unfortunate event. Likely if only one of these "holes" had been present, the error would not have occurred.

When errors like these do occur, it is important to talk about *why*. This should be done with the whole team and in a way that makes everyone feel safe to contribute. The error should be a shared responsibility, without focusing on shaming or blaming. In this way, a healthy and open discussion can generate recommendations (from all involved) to prevent the event from recurring. By involving everyone in a proper dialogue, each individual in the team will likely feel a responsibility to help reduce the likelihood of future errors.

Be aware of gaps not only in *your* knowledge and experience but also in your team members' knowledge and experience. This is crucial in a team setting to minimize episodes of disaster. If you don't recognize the holes, you won't be able to compensate for them. Be cognizant of when new variables are in play, and take steps to ensure that they do not have downstream consequences. Work hard to keep the holes in your Swiss cheese as small as possible and to prevent them from overlapping.

WHAT IF...?

I WAS A SECOND-YEAR resident when one of my mentors, Dr. Karim Damji, gave advice that has stayed with me through the years. He told us that "the mental preparation prior to surgery is just as important for the patient's outcome as the surgery itself." He encouraged us to visualize ourselves performing the surgery the day before. This meant taking the time to contemplate each step and anticipate what challenges we might face; to think about the case's unique aspects and what precautions might be necessary; to mentally go through the steps we would need to take to prevent complications and handle them if they occurred; and to imagine a worst-case scenario and our response.

In fact, it is good practice to do every surgery *three* times—first, the night before, in your mind; second, during the actual surgery; and third, afterward, by going over the surgery and breaking down what could have been improved upon. Many surgeons film every one of their surgeries so that if something non-routine happens, it can be reviewed. Try watching the videos of your surgeries as if you were watching someone else operating. How would you critique the surgery? How is the economy of movements? What could be improved?

The OR is different than the clinic, as decisions in the OR generally have to be made in a much more immediate and definitive way. Each step of surgery—from proper draping to closing up—builds on the last. Having an issue with one step often makes the next steps more difficult. The longer the surgery takes, the more likely it is that a patient under local anesthesia will start to get uncomfortable and uncooperative. As your hands and mind become fatigued, the risk of making errors increases. When the pressure is on, having a plan for various, less commonly encountered scenarios helps you be prepared to respond in a calmer, safer, and more organized fashion.

Throughout residency and fellowship, I would write out notes on every surgery. I would also ask myself "what if" questions and then list all the things I could do to prevent a given issue and what I could try iteratively to fix it. I knew that if plan A didn't work, there were still twenty-five letters left in the alphabet! *What if the posterior capsule ruptures during cataract surgery? What if a suprachoroidal hemorrhage occurs intraoperatively? What if there's an iris prolapse and I can't reduce it? What if I encounter an intraoperative malignant glaucoma?* Think through what you would do in these situations. Ask your mentors how they would handle them. Watch videos of how other surgeons manage these complications. You do not want to show up to the rodeo without a saddle, so to speak.

In the OR, adopt the Scout Motto and "be prepared!"

THE ACTIVE OBSERVER

DURING TRAINING, THE most instructive moments often involve you trying and failing at something, and then ceding the surgeon's seat to your attending. Watching how someone else successfully accomplishes a step is so much more meaningful right after you have struggled and been unable to do it. In these moments, you are *actively* observing and consciously reflecting on what you are seeing.

Remember when you were a medical student watching cataract surgery and didn't really appreciate a lot of the details? Then as a junior resident, you grasped the main concepts, but the subtleties of movements or positioning evaded you. Commit to being an active observer throughout your training. This is not easy. When you are at the sidescope, it is common to zone out and passively watch what is happening without actively thinking about it. Too often our minds get lazy and go into autopilot when someone else is doing the work. Instead, train yourself to watch while asking yourself questions like these: *How would I approach this? How are his hands positioned? How is she holding the instruments? Where has she placed her incisions? What machine settings is he using? How much force is she applying to the tissues? What angle of approach is he taking with his instruments?*

I remember during the first vitrectomies of my vitreoretinal fellowship, I was having difficulty lighting vitreous that was directly under the port that was holding the light pipe. When my attending and I switched chairs and I observed his hand position from outside of the microscope, I realized that my hand needed to direct the instrument almost perpendicular to the floor. Then I understood. Although I had seen him do this many times, I had not internalized it because I had not myself struggled with the movement.

Early (and often) in your training, remind yourself to tune in. There is a lot that can be learned by watching, and even more when you're actively observing.

DON'T TAKE
THE REPORT AS GOSPEL

"**H**MM. NORMAL MRI." I was working in the neuro-ophthalmology clinic as a fourth-year resident. My attending, Dr. Vivek Patel, had just finished his critical analysis of a radiology report. Mr. S., our patient, was carrying a diagnosis of normal tension glaucoma (NTG). He'd been referred to us to ensure there was no other cause for the progressive changes noted on his visual field tests. The MRI had been carried out primarily to rule out a tumor compressing the optic nerve. To me, it seemed like a pretty open-and-shut case. No tumor, so no worries; diagnosis of NTG confirmed.

Something, however, did not sit well with Dr. Patel. Yes, there was no mass, but what about that vessel? "Look at the nerves and look at that carotid artery," he said to me. The prechiasmal optic nerves were deflected from their normal course on the MRI scan. The culprit? A dolichoectatic carotid artery! And interestingly, the more distorted nerve was on

---

NOTE Dolichoectatic is one of my favorite words in medicine and means elongation and distension! Of course, my number-one favorite word (in case you were wondering) is borborygmi—the rumbling or gurgling sound your stomach makes caused by the movement of gas in your intestines.

the same side as the eye with the more severe visual field loss. The neurosurgery service became involved and subsequently performed an operation to place Teflon between the artery and nerve to buffer the pulsations from the artery. The surgery was a success and the progression of the patient's visual field changes slowed.

In my medical career, this was one of my first real-life introductions to the notion that we should look at the results of any test with a healthy dose of skepticism.

Dr. Patel told me, "Make use of imaging and blood tests and consultations to guide you, but always remember that they can be wrong! You know your patient best. A scan is just a scan. Without the clinician overlaying all the data and transposing it onto the clinical presentation, the puzzle may not be solved."

During my residency, the chair of the department at the time, Dr. Steven Gilberg, an oculoplastic surgeon, conveyed a story that also drove home this point. His patient had been worked up by rheumatology several years prior and was given the diagnosis of Sjögren syndrome. Of note, blood tests for granulomatosis with polyangiitis (GPA) had been negative on separate occasions years apart. Dr. Gilberg saw the patient regarding new eyelid swelling, periocular pain, and, on CT scan imaging, enlarged lacrimal glands. He performed a biopsy, which demonstrated chronic granulomatous inflammation. One day the patient called and said, "Doctor, I have gone blind in both eyes, but don't worry it happened once before and it came back!" The patient had experienced an occlusion of the central retinal artery in each eye.[2] This unusual presentation

---

2 F. Costello, S. Gilberg, J. Karsh, B. Burns, and B. Leonard, "Bilateral Simultaneous Central Retinal Artery Occlusions in Wegener Granulomatosis," *Journal of Neuro-Ophthalmology* 25, no. 1 (2005): 29–32.

had been previously described in GPA, and the team of physicians involved in the patient's care were suspicious enough to reorder the test. You guessed it—this time it came back positive! The patient was given the correct diagnosis of limited GPA and started on appropriate treatment. So, if you really suspect a diagnosis and the tests are not supportive, sometimes it's worthwhile running the investigations again.

There is no perfect test. False positives and false negatives must always be a part of the conversation. Many investigations that you will order rely on the interpretation of another specialist, such as a radiologist or pathologist. As such, that individual's level of expertise and human error come into play. Take a second to look at who read the report. The junior radiology resident may not have as refined an interpretation as the seasoned attending. The general pathologist's assessment of sections of an intraocular mass may not be as accurate as that of the pathologist with fellowship training in ophthalmic pathology. Work with the very appropriate assumption that, from time to time, whatever test you order *will* yield an inaccurate result and could lead you astray.

This underscores the importance of resisting the temptation to order a barrage of tests willy-nilly. The uveitis literature has approached this concept in a sophisticated manner, employing the mathematical construct of Bayes' theorem.[3] When deciding whether or not to order a test, consider the sensitivity and specificity of the test as well as the pretest likelihood of the disease being present. If, for example, you believe that there's an extremely low chance that your patient's uveitis is caused by tuberculosis, most people would counsel you to

---

[3] J.T. Rosenbaum, and R. Wernick, "The utility of routine screening of patients with uveitis for systemic lupus erythematosus or tuberculosis. A Bayesian analysis," *Archives of Ophthalmology* 108, no. 9 (1990): 1291-1293.

not even order the test. Don't get stuck with the false positive, wishing you hadn't ordered the test!

There will be times in your career when a blood test you order to help diagnose a patient will come back as a false negative. There will be occasions when the imaging report you receive is incorrect. You will encounter situations in which the physician to whom you referred your patient makes a wrong assessment. Your patient may suffer if you have blind faith in the report.

So, order tests only when necessary, have a healthy skepticism for any results, and know what you intend to do with the information you receive.

PRACTICE MAKES PERMANENT

WHEN I WAS a kid, I had to play the oboe in the school band. I say I *had* to because, at the time, I felt I was unfairly forced to. If I am honest though, it was probably my own darn fault. Since *everybody* wanted to play the saxophone, each student had to write down their top-three preferred instruments, and then the band director would choose what you would play. I wrote down "#1 saxophone, #2 trumpet," and then (as a joke) "#3 oboe." I didn't even know what an oboe was! I was confident that if I didn't get my first choice, I would at least get my second and be playing the trumpet. However, as I was the only kid odd enough to write down oboe, the band director was thrilled and put me down for the instrument that, I would soon come to realize, made a sound resembling the call of a duck. I was crushed but, at the time, too timid and embarrassed to admit I had written it down as a joke.

Well, the best thing I took away from three years of oboe lessons was my teacher's mantra "Practice makes *permanent.*" I had always thought that practice made perfect. However, my teacher would regularly point out that, if indeed I was practicing (I was not), things were not becoming perfect. Her point was that if you practice something improperly again and again, it is going to become permanent technique. Practice does not necessarily make perfect—only practicing something perfectly will lead to this outcome!

As you are training, it is vital to identify good technique and to engrain this in your repertoire. Look around you and find clinicians and surgeons who are known to be exceptional, efficient, safe, and independent and strive to emulate them. When you are on your own, slow down and try to reproduce what you have seen them do. Go to the wet lab regularly. Videotape your movements and critique them. With repetition and reflection, good technique will become a permanent part of what you do!

THE INDEPENDENT SURGEON

"GIVE HIM A wrench and he can fix the retina." This was our scrub nurse's description of Dr. John Chen on my first day in the operating room during my fellowship. I watched with interest as he placed a scleral buckle without requiring any additional helping hands. (Looking back, I wonder if he hesitated asking me to assist because he sensed that his fresh, bright-eyed but inexperienced fellow would be more of an obstacle than anything.) He held two ties with his left hand to control the muscles, positioned a Q-Tip to retract the conjunctiva and Tenon's with his left-hand pinky finger, and then used his right hand to craft the scleral belt loops for the buckle. I have yet to see a more efficient and elegant approach to placing a scleral buckle.

In the operating room, it is advisable to be as adaptable and as independent as possible in order to increase your efficiency and decrease your reliance on others. Without the benefit of a skilled assistant, how would you perform intraoperative scleral depression? What about something as simple as watering the cornea during cataract surgery? If the machine has an error and you are working with an inexperienced staff member, would you know how to fix most problems? Have you taken the time to learn how to set up the cataract or vitrectomy machine? Or would you need to rely on those around you? You will not always have your most knowledgeable team around you.

Years ago, about once a month, I would perform cataract surgery in a small peripheral hospital. During one such visit, my first two OR days went smoothly, but on my third day in the OR, I unfortunately had a case in which the posterior capsule was compromised. Slowly and methodically, I was able to successfully remove all residual lens material and place a sulcus lens with optic capture. I stained with diluted triamcinolone to visualize if there was any vitreous present in the anterior chamber. Sure enough, there was a wick coming to the main wound! *No problem*, I said to myself. *A little vitrectomy and we'll be home free.* I calmly asked the nurses to set up the anterior vitrector. My request was met with a series of blank stares. They had never done it before! The patient was getting restless and, in the stress of the moment, I realized that neither had I. While the set-up ended up being relatively straightforward, I am sure it would have gone more smoothly and felt less nerve-wracking had I taken the time to learn how to do it beforehand.

Take the time to find out what is available to you and where everything is stocked in the OR. This is particularly important if you operate at multiple sites. Creating "cheat sheets" for the OR is a great idea to help guide the nurses as to your specific instrument preferences or set-ups for uncommon scenarios.

Do not rely on others to make sure that things go well. Be ready to take control and be independent.

PERFECT IS THE ENEMY OF GOOD

THE TITLE OF this chapter is a useful mantra to keep in mind in the operating room. Its essence is: don't risk creating a problem because 99 percent wasn't good enough.

Not pushing for perfect does not necessarily mean the patient's outcome will be compromised. Every move and decision you make has the potential for error. For example, in a challenging cataract surgery, if the risk of rupturing the posterior capsule seems high, leaving a small wisp of cortex may be a reasonable compromise. Or if, after peeling an epiretinal membrane during vitrectomy surgery, visualization has become an issue that cannot be easily resolved, not pushing forward to peel the ILM may be in the patient's best interest. Patients in such cases will still do well and will likely do better than if a complication had arisen.

In fact, after a complication, it is not uncommon for the surgeon to think, *I wish I hadn't pushed on. I wish I had just stopped there.* When the job is essentially done, make sure that the "icing on the cake" maneuvers do not undo your hard work and create further problems.

I like to call this the "shoes on a baby" concept. I have always found shoes on infants hilarious. While they may look cool, they serve absolutely no purpose for a kid who cannot walk. So if you are putting shoes on the baby, but you see it is going to make him cry, stop and just leave it! In touchy situations, the fuss is probably just not worth the fashion statement.

DON'T FIGHT YOURSELF

SURGERY CAN BE described as a pyramid, with each step dependent on the one before it. How successful you are with one step influences how challenging the next step will be. Everything from draping properly at the beginning of the case to taking the speculum out at the end requires vigilance and care. Do yourself a favor and make sure you always address the basics. Get a good night's sleep and eat something before your day begins. Take the time to adjust the stretcher, the patient's head, the pedals, your chair, and the microscope. Giving your patient your absolute best effort requires you to be, at the very least, alert, well fed, and comfortable.

Performing surgery, especially when you are in the early stages of your training, can be very stressful. So the last thing you want to do is make things harder for yourself than they need to be. It takes years (many!) of operating and reflecting to progressively increase one's confidence and skill level. After performing a certain number of surgical cases in your training, you may start to feel relatively comfortable in the OR. And then—*wham!*—a case comes along in which everything feels awkward and difficult. Often this is due to the patient's challenging orbit or intraocular anatomy. Other times, painfully, it's a result of issues that *you* have created in what should have been an otherwise easy case. Essentially you end up fighting yourself!

I can think of many instances during my cataract surgery training when a case became cumbersome thanks to me. There was the case of the ballooning conjunctiva secondary to my slightly posterior corneal incision. I felt like I was drowning in the pool of fluid collecting on the cornea that was distorting my view. My attending, like a lifeguard, came to my rescue. In another case, I experienced for the first time a very "pushy" eye with a significant amount of posterior pressure. When we switched chairs, my attending recognized that the cause of our troubles was that I had overtightened the speculum in this smaller orbit. Simply loosening it solved the issue. There were several times during my retina fellowship when the bulk of my struggles came from simply not positioning the patient's head well at the start of the case. And in some vitrectomy cases, I have learned that when placing my ports, the difference between "comfortable" and "awkward" is a few millimeters.

When you are in training, it is easy for your attending to jump in and correct your mistakes. But once you are on your own, will you be able to quickly recognize and address issues, rather than obstinately pushing through them? Surgeons who aren't thinking make cases more burdensome for themselves. Take a second to figure out the issue and fix it. If something didn't work the first time, think through what needs to change to allow you to have success. And if you don't believe me, take it from Einstein himself, who said, "The definition of insanity is doing the same thing over and over again, but expecting different results."

SHOOT FOR 100 PERCENT

IT IS SAID that disease presentations fall into one of four categories:

1 Common presentations of common diseases	2 Common presentations of uncommon diseases
3 Uncommon presentations of common diseases	4 Uncommon presentations of uncommon diseases

By definition, the majority of your practice will comprise of patients who fall into category 1. Throughout your career, however, you will have your fair share of cases in the other three categories. The key is identifying (consciously or unconsciously) which patients fit into which of the four quadrants. It is easy to get lulled into a routine with your regular flow of category 1 patients. When a category 4 comes along, will you be able to recognize it and set in motion the appropriate laboratory and diagnostic tests?

Practice with an inquisitive mind, regularly asking yourself if the patient in front of you is your "bread and butter," or maybe someone with something more uncommon. If you do not consider the possibility of the rare or unusual, you will never diagnose it. By closing off diagnostic options, you risk sentencing your patient to a delay in appropriate care.

How many patients in your practice may be living with the wrong diagnosis? Take a second to think about it. Perhaps you are remembering a case that you misdiagnosed initially and then, with time, correctly diagnosed. Perhaps there are currently patients in your care who have you scratching your head while you wait for their tests to come back. Could there also be patients whom you confidently diagnosed, perhaps incorrectly? Back to the question... How many patients in your practice may be living with the wrong diagnosis? Be honest with yourself—give it a number. Don't worry, you don't have to tell anyone else! But if your answer is not zero, consider how you can lower it.

Imagine your career as a math test. Imagine that every question has a correct answer. And imagine that every patient you see has a correct diagnosis (or diagnoses) to find. What percentage are you going to miss because you were tired, rushing, biased, not thinking broadly, or not up-to-date on the newest literature? As physicians, we have survived years of taking exams and receiving grades. With the hard, concrete feedback of a grade, you knew how many questions you got right and how many you got wrong.

The difference between when you studied something like organic chemistry (sorry if I am bringing back any painful memories!) and now that you are in medicine is the patient. Only you were affected by your performance in organic chemistry. However, every patient you see is depending on your ability, affability, and availability. If their pathology is above your diagnostic and knowledge-base threshold, they may be negatively impacted. You've gone from studying mainly for your own success to studying for success in your patients' health. That's a big responsibility. Now that you are out on your own, when it matters most, no one is correcting you, and no one is giving you a mark. Make sure that if you *were* getting a grade on your diagnostic accuracy, you'd be shooting for 100 percent.

EXCUSE ME FOR SAYING "OOPS!"

AS A MEDICAL student, I was assisting an oculoplastics attending for the first time in the operating room during a blepharoplasty surgery. I was a little nervous, as everything was new for me, and I wanted to make a good impression. At one point, while cutting a suture (with shaky, unrelaxed hands), I inadvertently left an end longer than I had intended. I reflexively muttered a quiet, but still audible, "Oops!" I felt the attending's eyes swing toward me in the silence that preceded the patient's very nervous echo of my exclamation. "Oops?!" she enquired in a trembling voice. I felt terrible as I listened to the attending reassure her that everything was fine and explain away my "oops."

When the case was over, the attending took the opportunity to mentor me on operating room etiquette. He said, "Put yourself in the patient's place. Hearing 'oops' might be a very disconcerting thing! Having surgery can be a nerve-wracking experience for many patients. Patients under a local anesthetic can hear anything and everything someone utters. They can hear us discuss, argue, ponder, swear, and sigh. In this OR, we don't say 'oops'; we say 'excuse me' instead."

"Oops" is a loaded word. It conveys to anyone listening that a careless error has taken place. And without the ability to see the magnitude of that error or to understand its implications in context, some patients might interpret this event as consequential and fixate on it, when in reality, as in the above example, it may not be important.

One way of minimizing patients' dissatisfaction is through appropriate informed consent and managing expectations prior to deciding *together* to move forward with surgery. However, as surgeons, we deal with the full spectrum of human personalities. Sometimes, despite our best efforts and even in the absence of complications, a patient might still be unsatisfied. It is this subset of patients who are most likely to relate any perceived deficiencies regarding their postsurgical state to the "oops"-equivalent event—even if that incident was irrelevant.

I had learned my lesson. Or at least partially. While I had internalized the importance of watching what *I* said for the benefit of the patient, the importance of managing all of the people *around* me in an emotionally charged environment was not yet completely engrained in me. Fast-forward a few years... I was now a junior resident examining a patient who had been referred for a retinal detachment. I had a very keen medical student joining me. When I examined the patient, I discovered a large choroidal melanoma, rather than a typical rhegmatogenous retinal detachment. Before I initiated a very difficult conversation with my patient, the medical student took a quick look. "Oh my God!" exclaimed the student, unable to contain his amazement. I cringed. Needless to say, this wasn't how I had planned to start the conversation with the patient.

We have a responsibility to protect the patient's emotional well-being not only from our own comments and body language but also from those of all other people in the room. It is our duty to discuss this concept with all members of the team so that they are aware of their responsibility and can act accordingly. Now I try to always remind keen medical students of the importance of being sensitive to the patient, even in light of their own enthusiasm in seeing interesting pathology for the first time.

LAST LINE OF DEFENSE

AS SPECIALISTS, we are the so-called last line of defense because, with our specific training and expertise, we are often the professionals best poised to determine what is at the root of the patient's symptoms. If our defense doesn't catch it, the disease has more time to mount its offense.

There are situations in which a patient presents with symptoms that we, as physicians, have difficulty explaining. In some cases, the disease is still in its early stages and has not yet manifested itself in an obvious way. Or perhaps what the patient is experiencing is something that modern medicine has not yet been able to easily characterize or identify. The one thing that all clinicians dread is missing something.

For these types of situations, I hold onto words of wisdom I internalized from a neuro-ophthalmology talk I attended as a resident: "If the patient says that something is wrong with their vision and you can't find anything to explain it, make sure you've ordered the field!"

Several years later, I found myself unsure of what to make of a very pleasant patient with nonspecific visual complaints. He was referred for possible central serous chorioretinopathy

(CSR). However, the symptoms that he had experienced over the past months were somewhat nebulous and his history was not classic for this disease. My clinical examination was unrevealing. I obtained a fluorescein angiogram, autofluorescence images, and a macular OCT. As I reviewed these, nothing jumped out at me. Remembering the lesson from my residency, I organized a visual field test and set a follow-up visit to reexamine him without dilating drops and to assess his optic nerve function. When the field crossed my desk several days later, I was thankful I had ordered it—there was a significant defect! I reviewed it with a general ophthalmology colleague who, again bringing me back to my residency days, helped me appreciate the junctional scotoma. This was, of course, very suggestive of an intracranial lesion. Urgent neuro-imaging was organized and revealed an ICA aneurysm that was pushing on his optic chiasm! When I went back to look at the OCT again, I could now see the subtle finding of retinal nerve fiber layer thinning. (An optic nerve OCT was later done and showed this finding clearly.) If I hadn't ordered the visual field and instead simply communicated to the referring doctor that there were no signs of CSR, who knows how long it would have taken for someone to find the patient's aneurysm.

There were two lessons for me. First, when in doubt, get a field! Second, while we may be referred cases that are outside of our expertise, we're *still* the patient's best defense. And as all the great coaches say—defense wins championships!

DON'T GET BALDERDASHED!

IN THE BOARD game Balderdash, an obscure word is read aloud. Each player then writes down a definition for the word with the hope that the other participants might mistake it for the true meaning. All definitions—ridiculous imposters and the real one—are presented. Each player thereafter takes a stab at identifying the dictionary definition. Here is a recent round we played:

Hodad (\ ˈhō͵dad \)
a. A symmetric pattern
b. In surfing, a loud obnoxious person who has never actually surfed
c. A person very prone to falls
d. A cable used to secure a harness during mountain climbing
e. The state of being confused or perplexed

(Can you guess the correct answer?)

NOTE You get three points if you picked the correct answer, which is (b). If you picked (c), you sent two points my way!

So, what does Balderdash have to do with seeing patients in clinic? Well, it struck me that the goal in both scenarios is to find the correct answer and avoid any distractors.

New-onset floaters is a common referral to the ophthalmology resident clinic. *Every* first-year resident knows to perform a meticulous examination in this scenario to rule out a retinal tear, but that's not to say they all know *how* to do it. I can vividly recall the days when the complex skill of scleral depression evaded me and seemed like voodoo (hang in there—you'll get it... eventually!).

I was a second-year resident in our emergency clinic. The next chart I picked up was a follow-up check for floaters. I looked over the note written by the resident who'd seen the patient last. "Diagnosis: posterior vitreous detachment (PVD). No retinal tear." *Maybe today is the day I figure out scleral depression*, I thought positively as I brought the patient in the room. It turned out it wasn't. As I silently coached myself that I'd get it next time, I mindlessly documented my examination, more or less recopying the last resident's note.

When my attending was ready for me, I reviewed the case with him. "PVD follow-up, no tears," I relayed. We entered the room and my attending proceeded to quickly double-check that everything lined up. There was one of those uncomfortable moments of prolonged silence that every resident is familiar with, in which an attending spends a longer time than you would expect examining your patient. *What did I miss?* I wondered uneasily.

"We're going to step out for a second to grab some paperwork and we'll be back to explain everything and answer all of your questions," my attending explained to the patient.

When we were out of earshot of the patient, the attending asked me, "What else can cause floaters?"

"Uveitis?" I offered after a few seconds of pondering.

"That's exactly right."

After reviewing what I had missed, I was given the opportunity to reexamine the patient to convince myself and burn the teaching point into my memory banks. At the end of the clinic, my attending asked me a very interesting question: "Why do you think you came to the wrong diagnosis?"

I wasn't sure how to answer.

"Were you biased by the last resident's note?" he asked me.

I reflected on this and realized that this was the case. When I sat down with the patient, I *expected* her to have a PVD without a tear. My mind was prepared to find exactly that. I was not actively searching for anything more and was unlikely to see anything else unless it was glaringly obvious. My attending's advice to me: "Assume that you are wrong and then work to convince yourself that you are not."

We need to be able to look at each patient with fresh eyes. There are a lot of smokescreens that can cloud our vision as we seek the correct diagnostic path. We may be lulled in the wrong direction by something written in the referring doctor's letter or by the story provided by a medical student or resident. The patient may be a poor historian, or anatomical red herrings may lead us astray. And, of course, we all have our own inherent biases that can take us down the wrong path.

My attending was sharp enough not to get fooled by the smokescreen that I'd created. Let's strive to be like him and not get "balderdashed."

DON'T FLIP-FLOP

EVERYONE CHANGES THEIR mind from time to time. However, if you are known to hem and haw, you may be a source of frustration for your patients, staff, colleagues, and trainees. Flip-flopping leads to inefficiency. Take, for example, the physician who asks her administrative assistant to cancel a list of patients and then, a few days later, decides she does in fact want to work that day. If this is a one-off, no one will make a big deal about it. However, patients and the assistant are likely to become annoyed if this is a regular occurrence. Creating additional work for your staff will reduce the overall efficiency of your office.

In the operating room, strive to be the surgeon who is clear, calm, organized, and decisive. If you are contemplating your next move, have the discussion in your mind, and only once you have made your decision, verbalize it to the team. Make an effort to not be known as the surgeon who routinely asks for something, cancels the request, and then asks for it again seconds later. Try not to be wasteful. Be aware of what you ask for and make sure you use it!

In the clinic, most patients want a doctor who (1) communicates well and (2) seems to really know what they are doing. Patients' confidence in you can break down quite quickly if they see you frequently changing your management plan or contradicting yourself. Make sure your chart clearly documents what you have discussed with your patient and which direction you have agreed to pursue. Otherwise, you may forget your discussion by the next follow-up. If you do not maintain the same line of thought for treatment, you risk losing the patient's trust.

Indecisiveness does not breed confidence!

PROVIDE ANESTHESIA UNTO OTHERS AS YOU WOULD HAVE IT PROVIDED UNTO YOURSELF

A S PHYSICIANS, WE are often overworked and tired. However, this should not serve as an excuse to work in haste—*particularly* when it comes to anesthetizing a patient for a procedure. Nobody likes pain. But this is especially true for the small group of patients who fall in the ninety-ninth percentile of pain intolerance. (Oddly, I find these are often the same people who volunteer that they have a very high level of pain tolerance.) Some have so much anxiety and stress about having something done to their eyes that it is almost a form of torture!

Fear of the unknown is one of the biggest drivers of apprehension in patients undergoing a procedure for the first time. Take your time when freezing or numbing the eye. Radiate a calm demeanor and be gentle in your approach. Employ the "vocal local"—use a soothing tone to encourage as much relaxation as possible. Deliver ample anesthesia and, importantly, allow enough time for it to take effect. Tell your patients what to expect and let them know what is going to happen next ("This next part will burn a little"). Keep talking to them throughout the procedure to let them know that everything is going well ("It's looking good—you're doing great"). Give them words of encouragement ("We're almost done. Hang in there"). Try to always convey the three Cs: calmness, confidence, and competence.

It is even more important to emanate an air of expertise if you are the type to regularly get comments such as "You don't look old enough to be doing this." Make sure you have everything that you need laid out before you bring the patient into the room. Do a mental dry run if the procedure is something that you have not done on your own many times, and double-check that you are not missing anything. It can be unnerving for the patient to watch you fumbling around looking for things, and any added anxiety will likely affect their level of anesthesia. Be proactive in identifying who might require more anesthesia. Think of the high myope who, during cataract surgery, may experience reverse pupillary block. Know that very inflamed eyes are more challenging to anesthetize. Modify your approach—perhaps the case that is usually topical should be a peribulbar block. Perhaps the one that is typically a peribulbar block should, in fact, be under general anesthesia.

If you take the exact same approach with every patient, it's unlikely you'll always provide a comfortable experience. Take more time and precautions with those who are more sensitive. If you don't, you may create very negative encounters for a select few. Worse still, because of these unfavorable experiences and the fear and anxiety they've suffered, some people may not return. These patients may actually forego treatment (and possibly lose vision) in favor of avoiding another traumatic experience. Everyone deserves to have as humane an experience as possible. Yes, for some patients, this may take more effort on your part, but isn't that what you would want for yourself?

So, the next time a patient is more sensitive than most and is challenging to anesthetize, do not be surprised. Remember they are simply one of your one-percenters. Take more time and "top them up." Convey the three Cs. Do not blame the patient. Be careful to not make comments that make them feel bad or ashamed just because they require more anesthetic than the average bear. Remember it's not their fault that their eye is sensitive! It is, however, *your* job to take care of them.

Finally, put yourself in your patients' shoes. Who knows, maybe one day *you*'ll be on the operating table and will need a gentler approach.

THE INDICATION FOR DOING <BLANK> IS HAVING IT CROSS YOUR MIND

WHEN IT COMES to the health and safety of our patients, the saying "better safe than sorry" applies wholly. So, in those instances in the clinic or the OR when you are waffling over ordering a test or asking for another instrument, do yourself (and your patient) a favor and just go ahead and get it.

An exchange I had with one of my favorite surgical mentors taught me this notion. I was a junior resident and it was my first day in the OR with Dr. Michael Myles. "Do you know what the indications for VisionBlue are?" he asked. I reflected for a second on past cataract cases in which I had seen the dye used to enhance visualization of the anterior capsule of the lens. He watched me ponder for a bit, then said, "Just *thinking* about it. That's the indication! If you ever catch yourself looking at the eye and contemplating, *Should I use VisionBlue?* just go ahead and use it! You'll be kicking yourself if you don't and then struggle later as a result."

This is a little bit of a generalization, of course, as every decision we make comes with advantages and disadvantages. Depending on the invasiveness of the intervention, more deliberation may be required.

Let's consider another example. While most cataract surgeries are performed under local anesthesia, perhaps you're worried that a particular patient might move around too much with just topical. You wonder if they may benefit from a peribulbar block or even a general anesthetic. *But you could probably get away with topical, couldn't you?* says the voice in the back of your head. And there *is* a high probability that you *could* get away with it without any issues. Of course, in the background, you are also balancing a more involved anesthetic plan's associated systemic risk to your patient and your responsibility to act as a responsible manager of resources and expenses for the healthcare system. (You couldn't justify doing *every* cataract patient under general anesthesia, for example.)

So, did the voice that said you could get away with topical come from a place in your heart that was concerned about these factors? Or did it come from a place in your head that wanted to avoid the extra time and organization required to offer the other forms of anesthesia? Alternatively, did it come from a place in your ego that shouted, *You are a slick surgeon! Don't be a wimp—you can do it!* Humans are hardwired for a "survival of the fittest" mentality, so these types of thoughts are normal. Simply having them does not make you a monster. But in order to stop yourself from acting on your Cro-Magnon predispositions, you must be able to recognize them when they creep up and then push them away.

Make sure your decisions are *always* guided by what is best for the patient in front of you. Don't allow either convenience or hubris to get in the way of good patient care. Take the extra time and use the resources needed to optimize each and every outcome.

BAD FORM

"YOU LOOK LIKE a small animal trying to make itself big to scare off predators," said my attending. Suddenly I was aware of how uncomfortably I was sitting. Halfway through the case in the OR, my posture had degenerated enough to warrant this comment. At that moment, my knees were hanging apart, my shoulders were pulled up to my ears, and my elbows were splayed out to the walls. My back was arched and my eyes were bulging with the intensity of the situation. If they had stuck some quills on me, I'd have probably looked like a porcupine ready to attack.

When you are deeply focused on the operation, it is easy to miss the signs that your body is tensing up. "Sit up straight and thereafter try to make yourself as small as possible" was the advice my attending offered. "Do not let your limbs hang out—keep them close to your body and stack your joints. Do your best to hold onto the instruments with the minimal force required. Routinely employing the 'death grip' will not help your joints in the long run."

Early in my fellowship days, I was still mastering the art of indirect laser. At the time, simply achieving a clear view of anterior pathology was challenging for me, let alone maintaining it while performing scleral depression on a potentially uncomfortable and uncooperative patient and focusing and delivering laser of appropriate intensity and distribution. Although working with one's view inverted does not come naturally to anyone, time would stand still in the laser room for me in those early days. I swear that sometimes I would take in our first patient of the morning, only to emerge hours later mystified by the fact that the sun had somehow gone down in the meantime.

To this day, I still remember a patient who presented during my early fellowship days with an anterior retinal tear. "Don't move. OK, that's perfect. Stay right there. Actually, maybe look a little more to the left. Great. Hold that there." My neck was craned, my back was twisted, and my hip was offset as only one leg was carrying my weight, with the other held over the laser pedal poised to fire. I struggled and struggled to complete the indirect laser. My eyes went dry and burned as I concentrated so hard that I forgot to blink. When I finished (a long time later), I was pleased with my treatment of the patient's tear, but my body was not pleased with my treatment of my own neck and back. During the procedure, I had fought through the discomfort I felt. Later when I got home, my neck was so stiff and sore that I ended up lying still in bed on a regular regimen of Advil, Tylenol, and ice for the next thirty-six hours.

Lesson learned. Listen to your body! If it is feeling uncomfortable doing what you are asking it to do, take a break, and, if possible, change it up.

As ophthalmologists, we are prone to workplace injury. Sometimes our work will be a literal pain in the neck! This reality stems from three issues: (1) the high volume of patients that we see, (2) the awkward positions we allow ourselves to hold for extended periods of time during an examination or treatment, and (3) the repetitive movements we make again and again and again.

Stretch and stay active. Keep reminding yourself of your posture and positioning. Ask yourself, *Am I in a neutral position? What do I need to shift in order to feel more comfortable? Which muscles are tense and contracting to hold what I am doing?* In a long OR case, watch the clock and, at regular intervals, take a break.

Don't allow your career to die young from your bad posture. That's bad form!

KEEP IT CLEAN

"*THANK* YOU!" SAID the patient emphatically. I had just entered the room and was in the process of sanitizing my hands. It took me a second to realize she was reacting favorably to my hand hygiene (and wasn't being sarcastic since I was running late). She went on to describe how she was convinced that she had contracted an infection during a visit at another hospital, where she had found the hygiene to be "less than ideal."

Studies show that "less than ideal" is unfortunately the norm. In fact, a systemic review showed that the median compliance with hand-hygiene guidelines hovered around only 40 percent.[4] Rates declined when the healthcare professional was busier (e.g., multitasking) or engaged in "dirtier" tasks (e.g., those involving body fluids). Notably, physicians were less compliant than nurses.

And yet we've known for a long time that hand-washing reduces transmission of infectious disease. Two stories from

---

4 V. Erasmus, T.J. Daha, H. Brug, et al., "Systematic Review of Studies on Compliance with Hand Hygiene Guidelines in Hospital Care," *Infection Control & Hospital Epidemiology* 31, no. 3 (2010): 283–294.

medical school have always fascinated and stuck with me: (1) the misfortunes of Phineas Gage, and (2) the brilliance and tragedy of Ignaz Semmelweis. While the latter relates to the topic at hand, we will have to save the story of Mr. Gage for another time. (See "If We Were All the Same, It'd Be a Boring World.")

In 1846, the maternal mortality rates due to puerperal fever at two Vienna maternity wards were considerably different.[5] Dr. Semmelweis worked on the ward with the higher mortality rate and was committed to finding the reason for this disparity. Using the scientific method, he ruled out potential causes one by one. The breakthrough came when a pathologist colleague pricked himself during an autopsy and subsequently showed signs of puerperal fever prior to passing away. Semmelweis came to the realization that perhaps medical students and physicians who performed autopsies were transferring something to their patients and causing their illnesses and deaths. The other ward only employed midwives, who did not perform autopsies; perhaps this could explain the difference in mortality, he thought. Upon instituting hand-washing practices with chlorinated lime, the mortality rate on Dr. Semmelweis's ward fell drastically to a level comparable to that in the midwives' ward.

Apparently, Ignaz Semmelweis was not a "people person" and rubbed many colleagues the wrong way. In large part because of this, his recommendations unfortunately were not heeded at the time. He was dismissed from his post at the hospital and years later was committed to an insane asylum, where he would die a bitter, sad, and lonely death.

---

5 World Health Organization Patient Safety, *WHO Guidelines on Hand Hygiene in Health Care: First Global Patient Safety Challenge. Clean Care Is Safer Care* (Geneva: World Health Organization, 2009).

Although we've known of the importance of hand hygiene since the mid-1800s, due to our busy days and our attention being constantly pulled in different directions, we are always at risk of it slipping our mind. So remember poor Ignaz Semmelweis (and all those women who died in childbirth) and do your best to wash up and keep it clean between *every* patient!

THE ONLY WAY TO NEVER HAVE SURGICAL COMPLICATIONS IS TO NEVER OPERATE

ACCEPT IT. COMPLICATIONS will happen. And if they haven't, you just haven't done enough cases.

Operating can be stressful. *Especially* when things are not going well. At times, it can feel like the walls are falling in on you. Your first posterior capsule rupture, performed alone as an attending, may be accompanied by feelings of panic, tachycardia, diaphoresis, and a sense of impending doom. You may look at your hand under the microscope and wonder why it is shaking so much. Slooooow down. Take a deep breath and calm down. Believe in yourself. You can do this.

Remember that others before you have experienced what you are now experiencing—you are not alone. The seasoned surgeons will tell you that they've seen every complication possible. This is not from watching online videos. It is from being in the operating room over the years and seeing that everything that can go wrong will go wrong at some point.

In the old days, complications were hidden from colleagues. There was an atmosphere of shame and blame associated with errors. This was not healthy for either physicians or patients. Happily, the environment is now more conducive to sharing information. Measures such as "morbidity and mortality rounds" have promoted the culture of discussion with the goal of improving patient care by establishing specific protocols and better approaches. Realize that every movement and every decision in the operating room have the potential for complications. Before they actually happen to us, we should strive to be mentally prepared to manage them. I firmly believe that great surgeons are those who work on *becoming* great. When you do encounter a complication, learn from it. Record videos of your cases and break them down. Ask yourself, *What could I have done better in this case?*

In surgery, you need a good heart, a good plan, good execution, and some good luck. As a mentor of mine once said, "Be humble. And in case you are not humble, just do more surgery... you'll get there."

SOUND INTENTIONS... BUT POOR PLANNING AND EXECUTION

WHEN SHE WAS five years old, my niece, wanting to make the family car look nicer, used a rock to draw pictures on it. "Sound intentions," my father said afterward, reviewing her work, "but poor planning and execution."

We all want to perform flawless surgery for every patient. However, despite our good intentions, if we do not plan properly and execute things well, the outcome may not be desirable.

Reviewing charts prior to surgery is a very helpful practice. By doing so, we can identify things to remember and plan how to address unique challenges in each case. For example, if a patient being seen for cataract surgery reports a previous trauma to that eye, write notes to yourself about being prepared for zonular issues and have a capsular tension ring nearby. Knowing the surgical plan in advance will make you more efficient and safe in the operating room.

I was once referred a pseudophakic man who had a chronic retinal detachment with a very obvious large tear inferiorly. However, the distribution of his subretinal fluid suggested that, by Lincoff's rules, there must have been an additional break superonasally. During my clinical examination, I was unable to locate it, so I made a very clear note to myself on the chart to meticulously hunt around intraoperatively. During his surgery, I was successful in identifying the superior break, but it did take me a significant amount of time to find it, as it was very small and challenging to visualize due to peripheral opacities in both his cornea and capsular bag. I could have easily missed this break if I hadn't been actively looking for it, and it would have likely led to a re-detachment.

We should always remember the burden that is placed on the patient and their family when we have to return to the operating room. This often includes lost time from work and other activities, frustration, and disappointment.

As physicians, one of the principles that we strive to uphold is to "do no harm." Be thorough in your surgical planning and execution; otherwise you may end up doing more harm than good.

2

PRACTICE MANAGEMENT AND CAREER PLANNING

"Improvement begins with I."
ANONYMOUS

COME ON TIME AND BRING COOKIES

IT IS NO secret that the best way to reach many people's hearts is through their stomachs. There is no quicker method of establishing a good rapport with another human being (including your colleagues) than by showing up with a coffee or something edible. It's shameless, but it works. In fact, it can often make up for glaring character flaws! It shows you took the time to think about and do something nice for others.

Another important way to connect with the people around you is to make an effort to learn their names. It's not always an easy thing to do, but people really appreciate it. We work with many people who speak different languages and have different backgrounds. We may find their names unusual or hard to wrap our English tongues around. Do not be afraid to ask someone to pronounce their name for you. And the next time you see them, if you still aren't sure, ask again! We all think, *Oh, I should know their name by now! It will be embarrassing to ask again.* Don't be embarrassed! They won't mind if they see you are making an effort to pronounce their name correctly. Think about how you would feel if someone constantly mispronounced your name; you'd be happy to help them get it right. Learn some tricks like repeating the name in your head several times, associating the name with something else to help you remember, or linking their face with the face of someone else who shares the same name but whom you've known for years.

Never forget that your success will not simply be due to how intelligent or hardworking you are but also to how well you get along with the team around you. Administrative assistants, nurses, fellows, technicians, attendings, residents, medical students, and patients can all have a huge influence over the trajectory of your day (and your career). If you have the team on your side, they will voluntarily go the extra mile for you and your practice. However, if you do not have their respect and regard, you may face some lonely uphill battles.

Remember all the wise things your mom said: play nicely with others; do unto others as you would have done unto yourself; don't be rude; if you don't have something nice to say, don't say anything at all. And be on time! Walking in late is an easy way to get into the bad books of those who value punctuality. If you have a habit of being tardy, make a conscious change in your life and aim to get everywhere fifteen minutes early, equipped with cookies!

PICK UP
THE PHONE

IN THIS DAY and age of social networking, talking on the phone has become amazingly obsolete. We simply work more efficiently through other means such as email and text. And yet nothing comforts a patient more than having their physician take the time to call them. Other physicians also generally appreciate speaking with you regarding a consult (as opposed to with the clerk at the front desk who is reading your chicken scratch). By speaking directly with the referring physician, you can often quickly resolve the issue. Speaking through two administrative assistants can sometimes be like broken telephone.

If the matter is urgent or if a patient is distressed or worried, instead of asking my staff to pass on a message, I make the call myself. I think the extra effort is important and worthwhile in these cases. Patients are so appreciative. Perhaps because they don't expect it. I worked with an attending who would call all of his patients the night before taking them into the operating room to see if they had any final questions. His patients were always very grateful for this.

I once had a patient I was quite worried about, who was not responding to any of my office's messages. I took it upon myself to call one day and the patient actually answered. I expressed my concern for her vision and tactfully inquired why she hadn't come for her follow-up appointment. She admitted that she was very scared and anxious. It only took a few minutes to convince her to come in. I was surprised! It was another lesson that communication is so important and that, with certain patients, we sometimes need to go the extra mile to save them from themselves.

In another instance, one of my staff members told me that a patient's family had canceled an appointment because the patient had passed away. I had seen this patient about a half dozen times over the past year. She had a great sense of humor and I had really enjoyed our interactions. I felt no obligation to call the family and express my condolences, but I simply wanted to. When I rang, her son really appreciated that I had reached out to him.

In a world where most of our communication is conveyed by words on a screen, hearing someone else's voice can make a person's day.

DON'T LEAVE ANYONE OUT

WHEN YOU RECEIVE a consult, remember that there are a number of parties involved whose interests need to be satisfied when your work is done—the referring physician, the patient (and their family or caregivers), and you. Although everyone shares the same goal of maximizing the health of the patient, each of these individuals may have very different concerns. Often the patient's chief complaint has nothing to do with the referring doctor's reason for consulting you. It is important to take the time to understand and address both. This is a concept we learned years ago in medical school but that sometimes slips our minds. If we just look at the referral letter and do not cater to the patients' concerns, they will leave our interactions dissatisfied. Of course, if we get lost in patients' grievances and forget about the specific questions posed by referring doctors, the latter likely will not be pleased and may consider referring elsewhere next time.

As the specialist, you will often find pathology that the referring physician did not note and that the patient is not aware of. For example, when I am referred a rhegmatogenous retinal detachment, it is not uncommon for me to find a previously undetected retinal break or small retinal detachment in the *fellow* eye! This is a lesson to not just focus on the reason for referral but to do a comprehensive examination as well. Yes, the patient has been sent in for a specific question by their doctor, and yes, the patient has their own particular concerns—but there is nothing more satisfying than attending to both of those concerns and then, on top of that, demonstrating your expertise by catching another problem before it negatively affects the patient. Make sure everyone involved feels heard—the referring doctor, the patient, and even the voice in your own head that asks if you have missed anything.

DO A SELF-AUDIT FROM TIME TO TIME

WHILE I WAS writing this book, our residency program was undergoing an internal review for accreditation. The internal review is a useful mechanism to ensure that a program is on the right track. As is typically the case, the external review will be done several years later, affording the department time to remedy weak areas prior to the main event.

It occurred to me that implementing a process like this for my own practice would have its benefits. Historically, physicians graduated from residency programs and, in general, were left to their own devices for quality-assurance purposes. But times have changed. Patients demand more accountability from their healthcare providers, and hospitals and regulatory bodies have followed suit. Some departments regularly audit physician charts for billing and documentation purposes, track patient satisfaction surveys, and review surgeon complication rates. In other cases, a doctor may only be subjected to an audit in the event of a complaint or secondary to irregular billing practices.

If your department does not have a scheduled review of charts, consider executing this for yourself. This is especially useful when you are new in a practice and are getting used to a different charting system or way of billing. Every so often, take a random selection of ten or twenty of your charts and critically appraise them with an outsider's eye. Think about completeness, consistency, clarity, contentiousness, common sense, communication, and complications. Better yet, ask an established colleague whom you trust for their feedback. Would they have done anything different in any specific case? Do they have any constructive criticism for you?

The growth of electronic medical records has facilitated data mining for a practice. Ask any question, and if the data are being inputted, you can output the answer. How many cases of new-onset exudative macular degeneration do you see per month? What is your posterior capsule rupture rate? At what stage in your patient's clinic visit do they spend the most time waiting?

Even more powerful data can be accessed through participation in clinical registries. By aggregating large volumes of data on patient outcomes and physician trends, national averages can be established. The American Academy of Ophthalmology created the Intelligent Research in Sight (IRIS) Registry to help ophthalmologists practicing in the United States better understand how their performance stacks up and continually achieve more for their patients.

It is human nature to shy away from critically evaluating one's own performance. We worry about the time it will take, and, even more so, we worry about what we will find—our errors, complications, and inadequacies. However, by being transparent with ourselves, we can find ways to work toward excellence and optimal patient care.

DOCUMENT WELL

WE ALL FIND documenting tedious and time-consuming. We wish we could just care for our patients and not worry about the associated paperwork clogging our day. And yet, for billing and insurance purposes, and for communicating with colleagues, we have to remember how extremely valuable documentation is.

Certainly, there are strategies to reduce the volume of paperwork in our practices. Many physicians employ scribes for recording data. In addition, most electronic medical record programs are able to generate automated letters to referring doctors, replacing the need to dictate.

That being said, the higher stakes the interaction, the more documentation you should have and the less automated it should appear to be to anyone critically evaluating it. If ever you are concerned about a patient interaction, document clearly what occurred from your point of view. In the unfortunate situation that your case undergoes an official review, your documentation will play a critical role as evidence of what happened. Remember that whatever you write in your chart may one day be accessed by the patient, their lawyers, or the insurance company. Take care, therefore, not to write something inflammatory about that patient who gets under your skin. Be mindful to always be respectful and professional in your records. Ask yourself, *If another specialist looks at my chart, would they feel it was appropriate?* In fact, if a patient requests a copy of their chart, they may indeed be doing it in order to get a second opinion.

In addition to planning for the worst-case scenarios in which your chart is audited for unpleasant reasons or your patient leaves your practice, consider documenting well to enhance others' perceptions of your approach. Some people do great work and yet unfortunately have poor communication with referring doctors. This may, over time, lead to a loss of consults and confidence. Referring doctors like timely, clear, informative reports. In straightforward cases, there is not much need for lengthy and overly detailed reports. However, in unusual or complicated cases, the manner in which details are described in your report is an opportunity to really impress.

During your training, take the time to internalize how your attendings dictate, document, and make notes. When you are at conferences, note how the experts interpret imaging and what questions they ask in difficult cases. Communicating ideas in a sophisticated and intelligent way is crucial in your interactions with colleagues and referring doctors. This requires gathering a lexicon of phrases, terms, and concepts and being able to relay them appropriately. There is a finite amount of pathology that will come across your desk, and it will present in a finite number of ways. So, aim to be able to describe pathology in a way that will impress others. As an attending of mine used to say, "Try picking out the details that other people would have missed."

WHO DO YOU THINK YOU'RE DEALING WITH?

"Oh, your husband works in the hospital," I said, making casual conversation with a new patient as I sat down to start examining her. "Yes," she replied, "he is the head of infection control." I met this statement with a "deer in the headlights" blank stare. I'm sure it was obvious to her that I was frantically searching my memory banks for evidence that I had washed my hands when I walked in the room. A few pregnant seconds passed. Then—thank God—washing hands memory found! "Interesting," I replied nonchalantly. I couldn't help myself, however, from taking another handful of alcohol sanitizer from the dispenser and slathering my hands.

Clearly, the consequences of forgetting to wash my hands with the wife of our hospital's head of infection control worried me more than the same indiscretion would with another patient. Was this appropriate? Maybe not, but it seems to be human nature to worry more when the consequences are dire. Most of us become more aware and detail-oriented in our interactions when the stakes are high.

Would you approach a patient differently if he were the husband of a colleague of yours? If you were examining a healthcare litigation lawyer, would this play on your mind at all? Would this knowledge influence your interaction somewhat? If your answer is no, congratulations, you are a robot. All of you humans out there, however, shouldn't be ashamed or embarrassed to say yes!

When you think about the scenarios above, what thoughts go through your head? Likely, it's important to you that every patient has an exceptional overall experience. You would probably want them to walk away thinking that you were pleasant, that you took your time, and that you were gentle in your examination. You would want them to say that you had explained things clearly and at a level that they could understand, and that they got all their questions answered. You would likely want them to describe you as respectful and empathetic.

This should always be our approach. We are, however, human. Most of us need to remind ourselves of these goals from time to time. Particularly when we are overworked and tired after a long on-call stretch! Although the patient you are seeing may not be *your* loved one, friend, or colleague, they are that person to somebody else. We should strive to treat everyone exceptionally and equally.

MINIMIZING PATIENT GRIEVANCES

IN THE LIFE of a physician, there is probably nothing more nerve-wracking, gut-wrenching, and mentally exhausting than receiving an official patient complaint. And remember that every patient you see is a potential lawsuit or complaint—whether warranted or not!

Most commonly, these grievances stem from ineffective communication between the medical team and the patient rather than gross negligence. However, there's a higher risk of the patient taking the extra step from being discontented to taking legal action if certain factors are in play.

When you approach a new patient encounter, quickly ask yourself the following:

1. What are their motives and goals for the meeting?
2. What assumptions and preconceived notions are they bringing to the table that may need to be addressed?
3. Does their vocation or connection to you generate an added layer of complexity or concern to the therapeutic relationship?

The more emotionally charged the encounter, the higher stakes the pathology, and the less aligned the patient's perspective is with yours, the higher the chance that you'll have an issue.

For visual people, here is a series of scales that show the spectrum of the patients you will see during your career. Where will your next one fall? If they are to the extreme right on most of these scales, be ready for the challenge!

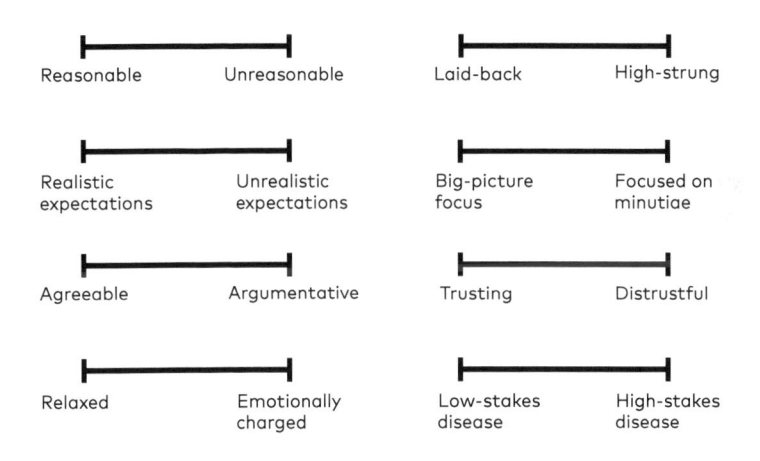

Reasonable — Unreasonable	Laid-back — High-strung
Realistic expectations — Unrealistic expectations	Big-picture focus — Focused on minutiae
Agreeable — Argumentative	Trusting — Distrustful
Relaxed — Emotionally charged	Low-stakes disease — High-stakes disease

Probably the most important question to ask yourself is *Where do they fall on the spectrum of reasonable to unreasonable?* Rule number one: don't fight with unreasonable—you will never win! Before the patient leaves your office, your goal should be to identify and bridge any disconnect or discordance between you. Not closing that gap will likely leave the patient dissatisfied. Frustrated patients whose needs are not met are more likely to lodge a complaint and seek satisfaction elsewhere. Check in with them at the conclusion of the interaction to ensure understanding. Ask them, "Does that sound reasonable?" This is a quick way to see if they are on board with what has been discussed or if they are unhappy and more time is required to address their concerns. Take the approach of "the customer is always right" and negotiate a mutually acceptable plan—you're smart enough to do that! Take the time to explain your recommendations regarding management and do not allow people to misconstrue your motives, interest or dedication to their care. Anyone who has been through a formal patient complaint—even if totally unfounded—knows it is not a fun process.

When you feel your "spidey sense" telling you that a certain patient interaction might be cause for concern, slooooow down. Be calm and think. Spend all the time you can ensuring that every question has been answered and document your interaction.

PRIVACY IS DEAD (AND THE INTERNET KILLED IT!)

IT IS SAID that there are only two certainties in this world: death and taxes. Well, I think it is time that we added a third truth to the list: the internet never forgets. Every Facebook post, Twitter retweet, or Instagram like is recorded for all of eternity, and data on literally every digital move you make are likely being collated and analyzed on some level.

Not only is your online privacy pretty much nonexistent, but we now live in an age where practically everyone carries around a video camera and audio recorder. You never know who might be filming you or when you might be on camera. Your next outburst or slipup may be the internet's next viral video! Before you know it, they will be auto-tuning your voice and making you YouTube famous!

These days every citizen is a news reporter ready to break a story—or, at the very least, embarrass someone. Our culture of shame is promoted by the anonymity that the web affords. You do not have to be in the wrong to be punished these days. Fake news, mob rules, and cyberbullying have become the new norm online, and victims are not infrequently condemned and sentenced without trial on the internet. No one said life would be fair.

Of course, in many cases, what is documented does tell the whole story. Take, for example, the case of an anesthesiologist whose disparaging comments regarding a patient were accidentally recorded by the patient's phone during his general anesthesia. The patient was awarded $500,000 in a lawsuit.

How secure are those emails you are sending? Be cognizant of how you express your thoughts. Before you send your message, read it over and make sure you would be comfortable in the event it got sent somewhere else. Someone can easily (whether purposefully or accidentally) forward what you have written and create an awkward or precarious situation for you.

Just as the carpenter measures twice and cuts once, with your online communications, read twice and post once.

EXTRA! EXTRA! READ ALL ABOUT IT!

WHEN WE WERE in medical school, my friends and I would regularly read with fascination the back pages of the magazine *Dialogue*. This publication from the College of Physicians and Surgeons of Ontario contained detailed descriptions of disciplinary hearings against physicians accused of unethical and wrongful behavior. We would marvel at how pathological these people were.

If you read enough issues of the magazine, certain themes emerged. There were the drug-dealing anesthesiologists ("one for me and one for you!"); the overworked emergency room doctors who became alcoholics; the burned-out orthopedic surgeons whose quality of work plummeted when they stopped giving a damn; the radiologists who overbilled services and inexplicably documented working on every single day of the 365-day calendar year. And, of course, in every issue, there was the psychiatrist who ventured too deep into the psychotherapy and fell in forbidden love with the patient.

Every physician dreads the prospect of receiving a disciplinary letter from their licensing body. But we knew that *we* would never be one of these stories. The individuals we read about were bad; they were flawed. They were *different* than the rest of us.

And then I read about someone I knew.

This was someone whom I respected and admired. I was conflicted. Were the statements about this person true? Could this be possible? Slowly my naïve view of "good and bad" in medicine and the world matured. I realized that, for the most part, these pages were not about bad people but about bad judgment calls. And that, in most cases, the people crossed the line when they were dealt a situation and simply succumbed to temptation. After they experienced no immediate negative consequences, the pattern of behavior became routine and further down the rabbit hole they went. The temptations in the more sensational cases—money, drugs, and sex—are those same temptations that can lead good people astray in any profession, relationship, or facet of life.

At the end of the day, your reputation is all you have. Be leery of excessive gifts from patients or pharmaceutical companies. Review your billing decisions with colleagues and ensure that they fit the norm and that you are not overbilling. Ask yourself, *If someone put this on a public forum for my family and friends to read, would I be OK with it?*

Keep temptations in check. Do not let a lapse in judgment in your next action or comment make you front-page news.

BE KIND TO YOUR COLLEAGUES

WHEN ANOTHER PHYSICIAN calls, they are asking for help. Remember that the physician who is referring to you does not, by definition, have your expertise or training. So, do not hold this over their head! You will need help one day too. Yes, not all consults are ideal. In fact, some make no sense whatsoever. But keep in mind that the referring physician has the same goal that you do: ensuring the health and safety of the patient. Take the time to educate your colleague and update them on the patient's evolution in a collegial way. If we complain about a "dumb" consult without making an effort to help prevent it from happening again, we simply contribute to the problem.

It is not uncommon for patients to come to us for a second opinion. Think twice before throwing others under the bus, so to speak. You were not present for the initial interaction, so you are getting a second-hand description of that encounter. We often only hear one side of the story (usually the patient's), which, of course, does not capture everything. In these scenarios, it's easy to be arrogant and to feed one's ego by looking down on someone else's work. Our natural tendency is to make assumptions that build ourselves up to be the hero and diminish the other by casting them as the villain in the story. Fight this tendency. While we always remember a better version of ourselves, we have in fact all been wrong before.

Be generous to others and give them the benefit of the doubt. Certainly, you owe it to the patient to be honest in your assessment. But tread carefully—focus on the facts and make sure that you are not making false assumptions and conclusions.

LET 'EM KNOW WHAT YOU WANT

WE HAVE EXPECTATIONS of those around us. When our expectations are not met, by either friends, family, or work colleagues, many of us take the path of least resistance: we grumble about it to someone else! Giving negative feedback can feel uncomfortable. This drives most of us to either avoid it completely, do a poor job of it, or gossip behind the person's back.

"Chris is never prepared for clinic."

"John is never dressed professionally."

"Susan is always late!"

Let's take a closer look at two scenarios. You have observed Susan, a new trainee, consistently arriving late for clinic. This frustrates you, as you are a stickler for punctuality. When speaking with one of your colleagues, you convey your disappointment in Susan's lack of professionalism. "Everyone else shows up on time. It is unacceptable for her to stroll in whenever she wants," you say. This continues until Susan's evaluation, when you finally give her the feedback that tardiness is unacceptable. When given the opportunity to speak, Susan says, "I honestly didn't realize it was a problem. I always get all my work done."

In this example, you assumed that all those around you shared and understood your expectations and values. In addition, when Susan fell short, you did not address this directly with her. Instead of discussing the situation and providing her with an earlier opportunity to align her behavior with your expectations, you allowed the trend to continue. You took a punitive approach at the time of evaluation, rather than a corrective approach by discussing it with her earlier. *Why didn't he tell me earlier?* Susan might have thought.

In scenario two, when Susan and the other new trainees start their rotation, you go through, one by one, the expectations that you have of them. You provide an opportunity for them to ask questions and to clarify issues. After the first week, you have a discreet discussion with Susan to understand why she has repeatedly come late to clinic. "Susan, when we initially discussed expectations for this rotation, I emphasized that I value being on time. Is there a reason why you have not been able to fulfil this commitment?"

Through this discussion, you learn that Susan and her family have gotten rid of one of their cars due to financial pressures. As a result, she has experienced challenges in getting to work on time. You convey that while you sympathize, you are interested in seeing her successfully organize her schedule so that she does not miss any more morning rounds.

In this scenario, you made expectations clear from the beginning, and a meeting took place with Susan *early* in order to (1) elicit and understand her perspective, (2) remind her of the expectations, and (3) give her an early opportunity to reevaluate how to meet expectations.

Too often we expect others to see things the way that we do. We presume they'll share our attitudes and preferences. Do not assume! Make your expectations clear in order to give people a chance to meet them. Know that giving (and receiving) negative feedback is often uncomfortable and does not come naturally for most of us. Always give feedback with the intention of helping the other person. Work on getting better at it, just like any other challenge.

DON'T JUST GO WITH THE FLOW— MANAGE IT!

I GLANCED DOWN at my watch as I exited the room. Thirty minutes behind schedule... and only the first patient on the list had been taken care of. I took a deep breath—it was going to be a long day.

This first referral of the day was a patient with a complicated history and challenging personality who was requesting a second opinion. This background was made clear in the consult letter, and it was obvious that the interaction would require an extended period of time. And yet when I'd triaged it, I had neglected to make a note for my booking team to under-book the morning accordingly. This lack of forethought had me moving on a treadmill at a pace I could never realistically keep up.

As I moved on to the next consult, I tried to block out the sea of patients' eyes shooting daggers at me from the waiting room. On top of a less-than-ideal start, the day was overbooked. "Thanks for your patience. I'm so sorry for your wait" became my catchphrase for the next nine hours. I skipped lunch and sealed off my bladder in a seemingly fruitless attempt to catch up. At the end of the marathon, I sat weary in my office. There was no one to blame but myself for the day's schedule. (Don't you hate when that happens? I mean, it's always nice when there is at least a medical student who can take the fall...)

Reality struck when I began working at my current practice and inherited many patients with chronic retinal pathologies who required injections. Unfortunately, in most cases, a single shot does not cure the patient's condition, but typically it can at least stabilize the disease for some time. As the drug only lasts a finite period in the eye, it is never long before a patient has to come back for an assessment and their next treatment. Medical retina physicians have thus become "injection-ologists." As I got accustomed to the layout and flow of my new practice, I found that I was extremely inefficient. It amazed me how little I could accomplish in so much time.

I needed ideas on how to improve my systems, so I asked a few colleagues and even traveled to a few clinics that were known to be efficient. I decided to try to understand and manage the flow. One colleague recommended a very instructive exercise: draw a "spaghetti diagram" to map out the actual flow of each person involved in the injection visit. The crisscrossing of both the patient and myself was amazing to see. At one of the clinics I visited, everything was organized with the goal of having the patient get from the start to the end of their visit taking the fewest number of steps. Their clinic's spaghetti diagram looked like a stick of uncooked pasta. Mine looked like a plate of cooked spaghetti tangled on itself.

A smooth clinical practice involves teamwork, so invest in the best office staff you possibly can. Remember these individuals will be the face of your practice! They are the ones who will often be called upon to de-escalate challenging patients on the phone or at the front desk. They will ensure your day-to-day operations run as efficiently as possible so that you can focus on your patients. Finally, consider hiring a consultant to review your typical week and give feedback on how you could improve your flow. They will help you identify rate-determining steps and clogs in the flow.

It pays to review your practice and to be actively involved in how your clinic and operating room days are organized. If you just "go with the flow," you will probably be inefficient most days, and some days you are just going to get creamed. So take control—instead of *going* with the flow, *know* the flow, and then *manage* the flow. By hiring the best staff and taking the time to review and reflect on all our practice processes, we can implement changes that increase efficiency, decrease our patients' wait times, and untangle some of the spaghetti.

FAST AND CARELESS LOSES THE RACE

WHEN WE WERE children, we all heard about "The Tortoise and the Hare" and how "slow and steady wins the race." But reflecting on Aesop's classic fable as an adult, I come to a slightly different moral: "fast and careless loses the race." Really, the tortoise's win was less about his own prowess and more about the hare's stupidity. The hare was positioned to blow the turtle out of the water! And what does he do? He takes a nap halfway through the race! And he doesn't even set an alarm. (At least set an alarm.) By the time the tortoise crossed the finish line, it was sundown. I would not call that a win. Slow and steady makes people ask why you have not finished yet.

During my retina fellowship, we would often see ninety patients in one clinic day. Initially, I was trying to see as many patients as quickly as I could. My attending saw that I was rushing through the day instead of taking the time to learn the craft. He sat me down one afternoon and told me, "Slow down. Learn more. Miss less." During training, if you have the opportunity to move slower, take advantage of it.

Certainly, when you are an attending, you cannot be a tortoise during clinic. Patients will get frustrated waiting, and longer days are not good for your back, your personal life, or your staff's morale. You will need to find a balance between speed and thoroughness. Rushing leads to mistakes, and mistakes take time to fix. As the hare's defeat taught us, if you want to win the race, you have to be both efficient *and* smart. For example, it is better to invest the time, attention, and diligence needed to remove that last piece of cortex safely than to rush and break the capsule and then be faced with decisions regarding the need for an anterior vitrectomy, sulcus lens placement, etc.

Maybe wise Aesop was trying to teach us a different moral: be the best of the tortoise *and* be the best of the hare. Seize every opportunity and don't forget to set an alarm!

FOOD FOR THOUGHT

WHAT MOTIVATES YOU to go to work every day? As ophthalmologists, we are fortunate to have a significant amount of variety in a typical workweek. Most of us have a mix of surgeries, lasers, minor procedures, and interesting new referrals that force us to stay sharp. In our field, the pace of evolution of imaging technologies and surgical and medical therapeutics is astounding. In addition to keeping up with the newest advances and literature, perhaps you are involved in research, teaching, advocacy, and/or administration. These can provide other levels of challenges, diversity, and meaning to a practice. And, of course, we routinely derive fulfillment and a sense of purpose from the appreciation expressed by our patients and their families for caring for their sight.

Now ask yourself what motivates the staff in your practice to go to work every day? While you get to be Sherlock Holmes, cracking *The Case of the Unwell Patient*, they often only get to see one small part of the story. As such, they may not always realize how valuable their efforts are in the overall care of the patient. Patients are more likely to express gratitude and appreciation to the physician rather than to the technician. Patients are also more likely to complain and be rude to support staff than to you! It is not hard to imagine that, despite carrying out important roles, your staff may be at risk of not feeling engaged in their work. What can you do to offer a more meaningful and fulfilling work environment? How can you create, and hopefully retain, a more involved team?

First, give them food for thought. I worked with a staff member during my training who would give a teaching session to his employees every six weeks over lunch. He would review cases and explain the diagnosis, prognosis, and treatment for the various pathologies that presented to the office. Watching this interaction was very instructive for me—I hadn't seen this done before in other practices! It was fascinating to witness the staff's level of interest and the questions they were asking. One of the technicians explained to me that these sessions put her work into perspective and gave it more purpose and meaning. Now she better appreciated how her contribution fit into the whole picture of treating the patient. Consider having staff attend events such as your local grand rounds, as well as select courses and conferences that will help grow their understanding of, and interest in, the practice.

Second, make sure they know they are valued and important members of the team. Seek their input. Ask them periodically how things are going. Get their advice about what could be improved. What are the worst parts of their jobs? Which parts of their jobs give them the most satisfaction? Never hesitate to pass on a genuine compliment if a staff member is performing at a high level and is good with patients. These small interactions with staff will go a long way in fostering a high level of job satisfaction.

THE CASE THAT GOT AWAY

IN RECENT YEARS, there has been an explosion in imaging in ophthalmology. Anterior segment surgeons make use of corneal topography, anterior segment optical coherence tomography (OCT), specular microscopy, and ultrasound biomicroscopy. Retina specialists take advantage of continuously evolving OCT technologies, fundus autofluorescence, and angiography with fluorescein and indocyanine green. Optic nerve OCTs and visual fields are routinely used in the field of glaucoma. Oculoplastic surgeons and neuro-ophthalmologists rely on CT and MRI and ultrasound. Securing high-quality and timely images affords you the opportunity to present, publish, and ponder.

During my fellowship, a patient with very unusual pathology came to us seeking a second opinion. He brought with him terrific images that had been taken elsewhere soon after the onset of his symptoms. The next day, I realized we hadn't kept a copy of his original pictures. Unfortunately, he did not show up for his follow-up appointment and, despite my best efforts, I was not able to reach him. Although we had reached a specific diagnosis, this case would have been very interesting to discuss with colleagues for other ideas and opinions.

Without the original images, however, the story would be incomplete. Describing what you saw to others is never as satisfying as showing them. In fact, sometimes they may identify details in the images that you hadn't noticed at the time.

This incident of the case that got away always reminds me to be proactive with acquiring imaging, lest I lose my chance. Sometimes the pathology evolves or resolves by the next visit. In some situations, one imaging modality may offer clues to the disease process, when others are less clear. A case of serpiginous choroiditis comes to mind in which only the fundus autofluorescence images really told the tale. In instances of very rare presentations (especially in areas outside of your subspecialty), you may not immediately recognize the diagnosis. Documenting the pathology's appearance at that moment in time with photography will give you the opportunity to ponder and reflect on the diagnosis and seek out other opinions, if need be.

Hence, it is useful to err on the side of obtaining as many images as possible (within the bounds of the resources available to you), particularly in very interesting, unusual, or instructive cases. If you want to publish the case, you can always decide *not* to use an image, but you may end up kicking yourself if you never took the photo.

Good images also come in handy for teaching sessions with medical students and residents, presentations for optometrists and ophthalmologists, conferences, and for posting on your website or in your office. As you go through your training and your career, take the time to index interesting images and cases. (Remember to get the patient's permission for the use of images where they could be personally identified.)

In one of my first months as a retina attending, I was asked to see an emergency patient with unilateral blurred vision. While the retina and vitreous were unremarkable, the patient's cornea had unusual changes that I had never seen before. Remembering the case that got away during my fellowship, I coordinated anterior segment photography and specular microscopy to document the pathology. After using various search terms to describe what I was seeing, I came across a few manuscripts discussing a rare condition that matched the patient's findings. While the pathology resolved relatively quickly, having the images from the day of presentation allowed me to obtain opinions from colleagues who specialized in diseases of the cornea. In addition, at the time there were only four manuscripts in the literature discussing this entity. Since we had high-quality images from the first visit through to resolution of the disease, we were able to submit the case for publication.

So remember, often a picture really is worth more than a thousand words.

DON'T BE
THE DINOSAUR

SOMEONE ONCE TOLD me, "Be careful about being the first person to use a new technology or therapeutic approach. But you also don't want to be the last one doing something proven to be safe and effective."

The pace of change in ophthalmology is incredible. In the recent past, cataract surgeons have witnessed the introduction of a host of new intraocular lenses, as well as a femtosecond laser. Novel approaches to fixating IOLs without capsular support, as well as artificial irises, have been described. The various corneal procedures that have evolved over time are a veritable alphabet soup: DSAEK, DMEK, DLK, K-PRO, LASIK, PRK, and PTK, just to name a few! Glaucoma surgeons now have a multitude of approaches available to them in the form of minimally invasive glaucoma surgery (MIGS), while every few years, retina surgeons adopt smaller-gauge instruments with faster cut rates.

There are likely things you do in your practice now that, in five years' time, you will be doing completely differently. Don't be left in the dust while others are forging ahead! Stay up to date. Go to meetings. Understand what new technologies, techniques, and treatments are on the horizon. Take the time to try them in a wet lab or learn more from people already using them in order to get a feel for whether they are worthwhile.

It is human nature to settle into a routine and not want to stretch outside of our comfort zone. While it is not easy, challenge yourself to be able to offer your patients the best standard of care available. When I joined an expert in endoscopic vitrectomy in his OR to learn more about the technique, he told me, "I never let myself get comfortable. I am always trying to improve and adapt, to find new and better ways of doing things."

Don't be a dinosaur—'cause we all know what happened to them.

YOU ONLY FIND WHAT YOU KNOW TO LOOK FOR

As a physician, you have great responsibility. Every patient comes to you with faith that you will identify their illness and provide them with appropriate care. Do not let your patient's clinical path be defined by what you didn't know or didn't do. If you're not sure about something, be humble enough to involve someone else who can help.

Having another person with a fresh perspective review the details of a case sometimes proves very fruitful. Two people can look at the same set of information and come away with vastly different insights. This is particularly true if there are differential levels of experience. Let me take you back to your histology sessions in medical school. Could you extract the same details from the slides as your teaching assistant or, for that matter, your professor? Of course not! However, the more you learned and the more experience you gained, the more you could see from those exact same slides.

In the old days, one's clinical and surgical growth after completing training was typically limited to learning from one's own cases and from periodic participation at conferences. Gone are the days when what was learned in residency would more or less last a career. Now we have instant access from any device to journals, clinical cases, comprehensive medical websites, surgical videos, expert opinions, online forums and debates, and live feeds from conferences. Today, from the comfort of our own homes, we can easily learn from someone halfway across the world.

There is so much material out there! Do yourself a favor and soak in as much as you can. Yes, it can be overwhelming, and no, you will never be able to read it all. But especially during your training years, commit to building a sound knowledge base. Read, read, read, and then read some more! Take some time out of each day, or at least each week, and make it a part of your routine. Speak with those senior to you and create a reading list of high-quality resources. Make a library of articles and index them well. Make specific and realistic goals for your reading and stick to them. Talk to colleagues and trade interesting cases. Get their opinions and see how they would approach things. All this will help you continue to expand your clinical and surgical acumen.

Push yourself to be better for your patients. Don't miss a diagnosis because you didn't know about it! Remember you only find what you know to look for.

FIND EFFICIENCIES FOR REPETITIVE TASKS

WITH AN AGING population, our healthcare system is becoming more and more strained, and physicians are seeing an increasing number of patients. Sometimes in our busy days, we become less communicative as we move through our patient encounters. Consider how much time you could gain in a day if you could shave just one minute off each patient interaction. However, while spending one minute less per patient might not affect the quality of medical care, the humanistic therapeutic patient-doctor relationship might suffer as a consequence. Are there other places where you can save time?

Retrieving this time from everything surrounding the patient-physician interaction, rather than by cutting short the actual patient encounter, should be a primary goal. In fact, by becoming more efficient, you will better serve your patients. Wait times will decrease and you will have more time to look each patient in the eyes—rather than losing time searching for forms or documenting your report.

Your overall efficiency is impacted by your office layout, the organization of equipment in your lanes, your charting system, and the number of technicians and staff members working alongside you. There are companies that specialize in assessing clinics and making suggestions for optimizing efficiency. Although these assessments are not cheap, they can be very worthwhile in the long run. But start with your own critical look at your current situation. An easy exercise is to think about your day and consider all the repetitive tasks you do. How could you reduce the time that you spend filling out forms and prescriptions, charting, eliciting information from patients, and conveying information in a meaningful way?

A useful concept to employ is the OHIO rule. Essentially, for each task that routinely comes across your desk, have a system for it that allows you to *only handle it once.*

I am willing to bet that only a handful of diagnoses make up the majority of your day-to-day practice. Hence, you could save time by having templates for your regular questions and examinations rather than (the extreme case of) writing everything out on a blank sheet of paper. Of course, electronic medical records have the *potential* to optimize efficiency for several of these tasks. Beware, however, that many EMR "solutions" out there actually *increase* the time it takes you to complete your notes! As well, if your room is not set up appropriately, patients spend most of their encounter with you looking at your head buried in the computer screen. In order to free themselves from charting, many doctors choose to hire a scribe, which (like anything else) has its advantages and disadvantages.

Consider offering patients an information sheet or a video that clearly explains (in accessible language) common diseases, their treatments, and the prognoses. Have a section that responds to frequently asked questions. Providing these materials has two immediate advantages for you and your patients. Patients get a clear explanation with details. They can take a handout away, mull it over, share it with their family, and not feel pressured to remember everything you said to them. And you save time by making a repetitive task more efficient. Thereafter, when you interact with the patient, they are already armed with the basics. You can tailor subsequent visits to address higher-level aspects that are unique to their case and personalize the information by, for example, showing them their diagnostic photographs. Hence, by eliminating time lost to performing repetitive tasks in your practice, you can in fact improve the *quality* of the patient encounter. Sure, a minority of patients will present with conditions that fall outside of the common diseases you see. However, if you can save time on the other 85 percent, you will be that much further ahead!

TWO THUMBS DOWN

I HAD JUST RECEIVED a terrible review online. I read it over and over again. My mind raced. I felt sick to my stomach. An overwhelming sadness filled me from head to toe. Who could the writer possibly be? I was so upset that someone had had a bad experience with me. *How could this have happened?* I asked myself. Was there anything I could do at this point to make things better? I stared at the screen. I had been criticized on a public forum. There it was for all time for anyone and everyone to see—colleagues, mentors, future patients, current patients, my family, my friends, residents, medical students, administrative assistants, nurses, and technicians. I felt ashamed and embarrassed.

I care deeply about my work. I can't stand not knowing something, and I am constantly challenging myself and others around me to stay up-to-date and informed. I obsess over details. The night before surgery, I often even dream about the finer points of the next day's list, as my subconscious fixates on how to minimize the risk of complications, particularly in more challenging cases.

I do my best to communicate well with patients and take the time to answer questions. I try to manage expectations and be realistic about outcomes. I recognize that most people only retain a percentage of the information we describe to them, so I provide them with a handout so that they can review the information again. I do not "convince" people to move forward with any specific treatment; I help each individual make a decision about what is best for them.

In medicine and surgery, there are times when our outcomes unfortunately do not meet our hopes and expectations for a patient. At least by working together, the patient and physician can explore all options to try to optimize the outcome. However, it is challenging to have that conversation when the issue is raised via an anonymous grievance online. This was probably the most frustrating part of my bad review: I felt powerless to help this individual. All we want as physicians is to try to provide the best care for our patients. That is our life's work. For the sake of my patient's health, I hoped that they would return for a follow-up and be open to having that discussion.

Knowing that I was not alone in getting a poor review helped me stay resilient in the days that followed. After speaking with various colleagues about this, I realized that it is not uncommon. Many people that I respect and admire had shared the same experience and associated emotions. Good physicians can get bad reviews. We shouldn't discount the negative comments and should do our best to incorporate changes to our practice to address any reasonable concerns. However, we should also not let them overwhelm us and prevent us from helping all the other patients who will benefit from our care.

Don't let the remarks left by the angry patient represent your "webutation." Those who have a negative experience are more likely to comment. Take control of your online reputation. Read the feedback and ask yourself if there could be truth to the negative comments. Perhaps your wait times *are* too long. How can you fix that? More and more patients go online to read about their doctor. Google yourself and see what they are seeing. Do good work and it will drown out the discontented minority.

SOAK IN THE BUSINESS

WHEN IT COMES to a "business sense," most physicians are seriously lacking. This shouldn't be a surprise; the majority of our time on the never-ending road to finishing training is dedicated to trying to cram in every last bit of medical knowledge. This leaves very little time for anything else (except for wishing we had more time to sleep!). We have hemorrhaged money to pay for our education and are so familiar with our debt that it feels like an unwelcome houseguest who shows no signs of leaving anytime soon.

Underlying all of this is the fact that most of us decided to pursue medicine primarily out of a desire to help others. Most physicians joined the profession to treat patients, not to run a business. And yet, for so many of us, the business side of medicine—the part for which we are least prepared—ends up consuming significant portions of our time, energy, and attention.

Not long ago, a colleague said to me, "I have spent more time in the past year studying building codes and permits, and rules around hiring and firing, than reading journal articles!"

You need to accept that there is a distinct possibility that at the end of your training, you will find yourself running a business. While we would all like to simply focus on our patients and keep up-to-date on the medical and surgical advancements in our specialty, it would be challenging to completely insulate ourselves from the business side of medicine. Certainly, if you have a totally academic practice and are salaried, there is much less to think about. However, those of us in private practice will have to make challenging business decisions along the way.

Good patient care is difficult to provide without excellent office staff, up-to-date equipment, and good facilities. All of these things cost money. To put it plainly, you can't offer your patients good care if your practice is bankrupt!

Take time in your last year of training to discuss the business side of medicine with your attendings and mentors. Get to know the billing codes well. Understand when it is appropriate to use which ones and when it is not. Otherwise, you will not get properly paid for your hard work and services! Get a sense of how to run an office and build its brand. Understand the salary scales of technicians and secretaries and the costs of various machines and equipment. Do your mentors have a business plan? What about a mission statement? What makes for an efficient office layout? Just as you probably have a folder for good medical articles that you want to refer back to, create one on practice management.

Instances will arise in which you will have to make the difficult decision on whether or not to charge a patient for your services. Insurance companies and governments have seen healthcare budgets explode. Increasingly, they are placing the burden on the physician's back to either eat the cost or be the bad guy and charge the patient for services that are not covered. This is a very frustrating proposition for most doctors. No one feels fairly treated when they are not compensated for work they provided. And yet putting money into the equation can place a strain on the physician-patient relationship. This, however, is a reality that you will likely have to face.

So will you charge patients for the lost income you incur from missed appointments? Will you fill out mountains of insurance forms and "sick notes" without being reimbursed for your time? What about noninsured services that are considered by your specialty as standard of care and medically necessary but fall outside of patients' coverage?

Through it all, always remember why you entered medicine. No matter how you approach the business side of medicine, make sure your primary focus remains the business of helping people.

TAKE TIME TO TEACH

THINK OF ALL the people over the years who were involved in your training. You surely had some amazing teachers who helped you get where you are today. Never forget this—give back and pay it forward!

Having trainees with you can slow you down, confound you at times, and squeeze your coronary arteries when their good intentions for patient care threaten to slide the situation out of the "safe zone." You likely can remember examples of doing all of these things to your mentors in days gone by.

Teaching takes patience. Surgical teaching takes patience and courage. And it takes trust: between the surgeon and learner, between the surgeon and patient, and between the patient and learner.

I almost made my attending fall out of his chair during one of my first cataract cases. It was only the second time I had ever made an incision into a live human eye in a real-life patient. Mrs. A. had consented for me to perform her surgery and I desperately wanted everything to go well. My heart was pounding. My focus was so intense that my eyelids refused to blink; my corneas burned and screamed for moisture. I'm surprised that I didn't pass out from holding my breath. Although not by intention, every movement I made was in slow motion—like I was a fly swimming in molasses. Slooooowly I brought the blade toward the cornea to carefully and meticulously craft the main incision. Suddenly, *wham!* I saw the knife fly like a bullet through the cornea, halfway across the anterior chamber, and come back out of the eye as quickly as it had gone in. My attending's gaze whipped up from the sidescope oculars and he stared at me dumbfounded. I was still trying to piece together what the heck had happened, when I saw the patient's hand move again under the drapes.

"Are you OK, Mrs. A.?" my attending asked. "We'll ask you to please not move and to keep your hands down by your side."

"Yes, sorry—it's just that my nose is so itchy!"

Mrs. A.'s hand had come up to scratch her nose and smacked my hand just as I was about to make the incision! This was the reason for the heavy-handed and swift technique I had involuntarily demonstrated.

Lesson: the longer you take to do something, the longer the patient has to become uncomfortable or fidget and move around. And, of course, we are always slower when we are training.

After we got Mrs. A. comfortable and reassessed the situation, the wound was noted to be slightly large but still manageable. I fully expected at this point to be given the curtain call and for my attending to switch spots with me. On the contrary, he asked me, "Are you OK to keep going?"

Medicine is an apprenticeship that survives only thanks to generous and caring teachers who can help us learn the craft in slow increments that are safe for both the patient and the trainee. My attending later explained to me, "Complications *can* happen and *will* happen in *everyone's* hands. Deviations from 'perfect' happen by situation, not by intention. I had confidence in you. And I wanted to make sure, that in this critical and potentially nerve-wracking moment, you had confidence in yourself too."

Teaching can be overwhelming at first. However, like anything, you will improve with practice, reflection, and hard work. What you feel comfortable teaching today likely will grow and expand and evolve over time. This is especially true for surgery. Remember that any time someone is observing you, you are in fact teaching—whether you're doing a good job of it or not!

Know that you cannot teach everything in one day, one clinic, or even one week. Be realistic: aim to transfer *at least* one concrete learning point from every teacher-learner experience. I worked with an attending who had this goal. At the end of each day, he would have us tell him the one take-home point we had learned. In this way, we would always leave with something tangible.

If you can find no other motivation to teach, just do it for selfish reasons—when you are old and gray and falling apart, you may need your students' care!

WHAT DO *YOU* THINK?

ONE DAY IN my second year of residency, I found myself in the glaucoma subspecialty clinic. Dr. Karim Damji, the attending and one of the editors of the bible of glaucoma (*Shields Textbook of Glaucoma*), asked me my thoughts on the treatment plan.

"So what do you think? What would you do in this case?"

By this stage in my medical career, I was used to being asked pop-quiz-type questions on the spot. "Pimping" trainees, as it is crassly called, is as much a part of medicine as the white coat. It serves as an informal way for attendings to evaluate students. The fear of public shame in incorrectly answering a question kept us working fiercely hard to build our knowledge base. In most cases, the questions were fair and were asked in the spirit of educating. However, everyone also experienced those attendings who enjoyed pimping to intimidate trainees and to highlight and enforce the hierarchy of medicine.

The manner in which Dr. Damji asked this question made me pause for a second. *Is he pimping me—or is he actually asking my opinion?* As the conversation continued, it became clear that he was genuinely interested in my thoughts on management and sincerely valued my opinion. This was not something I commonly experienced in my attending-trainee interactions. Here was a world-renowned specialist who was light-years ahead of me in training and experience, and he was respectfully engaging me (a junior resident) to see what I could contribute. (As it turns out, I was not able to contribute much, but that is beside the point!)

On my path to becoming an independent practitioner, and now as the attending who is asking the questions, I have always tried to remember the way Dr. Damji and other such mentors interacted with me. They made me understand that no matter what stage I was at and how knowledgeable I had become, it would be a mistake for me not to see what those around me had to teach me. This, of course, goes not just for other physicians but also other healthcare professionals. There were certainly many times during my fellowship and first years of practice when advice from an amazing scrub nurse made my life easier in the OR.

In the hierarchy of medicine, sometimes we physicians buy into the delusion that we are at the top of a pyramid. Do not fall into this trap. Remember that we are all valued members of a team who bring expertise in our common goal of helping our patients. Sometimes all it takes is asking, "What do you think?"

We should, of course, offer the same respect and consideration to our patients. Asking them "What do *you* think?" will often reveal assumptions or misconceptions that would benefit from discussion before we go over management options together. It may also encourage them to divulge important information that they otherwise might hold back for whatever reason (perhaps they're embarrassed, nervous, skeptical, etc.). This simple question empowers the person being asked—no matter who they are—and builds trust in the relationship.

CONFLICTED ABOUT YOUR INTERESTS?

THERE COMES A time in every physician's career when they need to consciously decide what their relationship with the pharmaceutical/medical device industry is going to look like. This is a serious topic that often polarizes people and offers many pitfalls if you are not careful. So, first, let's jump right to the two most important facts to remember.

FACT #1: *Any* interaction you have with industry has an influence on you.

Plain and simple. There is ample evidence in the literature that this is the case. If you think otherwise, you're fooling yourself. If companies' marketing efforts were not good for their bottom line, they would not be spending billions of dollars each year to this end. Interestingly, most physicians, when asked, believe that they can remain objective but suspect that the judgement of their colleagues is more easily clouded.[6]

---

6 S. Chimonas, T. A. Brennan, and D. J. Rothman, "Physicians and Drug Representatives: Exploring the Dynamics of the Relationship" *Journal of General Internal Medicine* 22, no. 2 (2007): 184-190.

FACT #2: You are a matchmaker, and every company wants to sell you on how their product would be perfect for your patient.

Let's remind ourselves about the fundamental difference between your position and that of industry. You have been entrusted by your patients with the privilege to care for them in their vulnerable time of illness. You have a duty to care for them in an altruistic and empathetic way and to protect them from harm. There is an expectation that you will not abuse your power and that you will provide an unbiased overview of their options and help each patient decide what would be best for them.

While you, as the physician, focus on the *patient* and consider *all* options out there, each company is understandably married to its own product and does its best to convince you that it's the best for your patients.

From the pharmaceutical or medical device company's perspective, it has spent a substantial amount of time, money, resources, and risk into getting the product from idea to marketplace. And for every product that makes it, there are probably fifty others that do not. So, each company is heavily invested in anything that overcomes the many hurdles and satisfies the numerous standards, tests, and regulations along the way. Therefore, there is a lot of pressure to sell this product. After all, a company that doesn't make money won't survive. It may be in the business of healthcare, but to remain in healthcare, it has to first and foremost stay in business! So the company researches and formulates strategies to market its drug or device and finds every angle to promote it and put it on your radar. It will hire likeable representatives to meet with you with the hope that you'll enjoy spending time with them. The rep will show you all the data and information that presents their product in a good light. They will try to dispel, downplay, or justify any negative information that has come out about their product. And when you meet a competitor's rep, they will walk you along a similar path but give you their perspective instead. When there are multiple companies with similar products in the same sphere, you feel like you're hosting a debate and watching the development of the most convincing arguments.

Some of the information companies use is accurate and reliable. In other cases, they may present you with softer and more biased data that really just amount to sophisticated marketing. Therefore, you have to be exceptionally good at critically appraising the information that is being presented to you. Know how to spot the biases and maintain a healthy skepticism. Most of what industry presents has some merit and doesn't have to be discounted completely, but you must always consider the source and take any information with a grain of salt. If anyone gets creative enough with the numbers, they're bound to find something that supports their product. (Remember the old joke: statistics are accurate and reliable in only 87 percent of cases, and in the other 19 percent, they are totally off.)

By this point, you might be thinking to yourself, *This guy is totally anti-pharma.* I'm not. I have consulted for multiple companies, given talks, and attended lots of industry-sponsored continuing medical education (CME) dinners. But I am conflicted at times. And before diving in, I always ask myself whether what I am signing up for seems appropriate.

There are positives to engaging with industry. For example, it's a boon to be able to secure free samples for patients who do not have coverage for the treatment. Clinical trials are very expensive and, in an age when government research funding has dried up, many companies have stepped in to fill the void. Industry-sponsored research, with all the caveats and potential biases that might come with it, can be very instructive. In addition, the CME events that focus less on marketing and provide a forum for candid and honest discussions can be very informative. Partnerships between physicians and industry to develop new instrumentation and drugs are how our field evolves to improve patient care. Having physicians involved in this process is essential to ensure that the products our patients need will be available. Finally, many physicians are innovators and they need industry to bring their solutions for improved patient care to market.

When interacting with pharma, take a second to ask yourself, *What is my motivation here?* If your answer resembles anything from the above paragraph, you may be doing it for the right reasons. If, on the other hand, you find yourself harboring thoughts about "easy money," "lavish dinners," or "prestige from being at the podium and building your brand," your actions may be solely for self-promotion and personal gain. If so, it's time to tread carefully.

You are an expert in your field. You have a sphere of influence with your colleagues, referring doctors, and the public in general. You therefore hold significant value to the pharmaceutical companies. Remember if you speak at a company's event, in a way you are giving it your endorsement. So, as you can imagine, you won't likely encounter obstacles to getting on the podium to speak. The challenge for you will be determining whether you want to be there or not, and whether you deem it to be an appropriate opportunity.

If you are giving a talk, take the time to clearly understand how much leeway you have. Will you have free license to speak on whatever topic you like? Or have you been hired to essentially market and promote a product? Will you be able to convey your actual experience with the product or will any negative comments be censored? Are you restricted to only using slides that the company has created? Do you believe in what you are saying?

Many physicians recommend keeping industry at arm's length to prevent any conflict of interest. You may come to that conclusion yourself. However, if you see value in partnering with industry, hopefully it is to benefit your patients and profession, rather than you personally. Be cognizant of how you conduct yourself and what is considered acceptable practice. Your university or licensing body may have a policy statement on this. A few good resources for physicians practicing in Canada include the Royal College of Physicians and Surgeons[7] and the Canadian Medical Association.[8]

Physician-industry relationships are a complex issue and you will have to decide what your own comfort level is. Evaluate each request and opportunity carefully. Remember, at the end of the day, your name and reputation are your most valuable assets, so take good care of them.

---

7 Jeff Blackmer, "Relationships Between Physicians and Industry," Royal College of Physicians and Surgeons of Canada. Available at www.royalcollege.ca/rcsite/documents/bioethics/relationships-between-physicians-industry-e.pdf.

8 Canadian Medical Association, "CMA Policy: Guidelines for Physicians in Interactions with Industry." Available at policybase.cma.ca/dbtw-wpd/Policypdf/PD08-01.pdf.

SOMETIMES YOU GOTTA BE THE BAD GUY

"I'M READY and willing, doc!" Mr. L. was all smiles as he saw me approaching; his turn had *finally* come. I returned the smile. I always feel so bad for our patients as they wait for surgery. We ask them to come early so we can give them a funny gown to wear, and then we drown their eye in drops that burn and blur. "Now that I'm starved, bored, and tired, I think I deserve to go in!" Mr. L. exclaimed. I chuckled and gave Mr. L. an empathetic smile. "Yes, you're up next! And you'll be happy to know that in addition to making you starved, bored, and tired, we decided we'll freeze you as well. The OR is pretty darn chilly, and everything we've got in there for you is either cold or stingy!" I joked as we entered the room. Our circulating nurse brought Mr. L. a warm blanket as we began our preoperative surgical checklist.

"Doc, I should tell you one thing," said Mr. L.

"What's that?" I asked.

"I've been having a lot of tearing out of the eye we're going to do today. It got really bad about a month ago, and now, every day, the tears just roll down my face all day. I just thought I'd tell you."

Canceling a surgery is never fun. The lost OR time is hard for the surgeon to swallow. For the poor patient, it means another day off work and reorganizing schedules with family and friends. The prospect of getting back to regular life is again further delayed while surgery is rescheduled. Probably worst of all, however, it means coming back for another day of being starved, bored, and tired! How disappointing.

"Mr. L., I am very concerned that your tear duct might be blocked. This can put you at a higher risk for an infection. I am truly sorry, but I think we should postpone your surgery. I know this is very frustrating. I know how challenging it can be to get organized for the surgery and I know you'd probably like to just get it over with. However, I think it would be safest if we looked into this tearing thing first and then found another date for surgery."

It took a little convincing, but with the help of the nursing and anesthesia teams, I was able to persuade Mr. L. that we had his best interests at heart and that it was important to reschedule. This was the first time I had canceled someone's surgery. Although I knew that I had done the right thing, immediately afterward, I had a very dissatisfied feeling. I had been forced to disappoint someone I cared about because I was worried for his safety and felt I knew what was best for him... it dawned on me that I was officially ready to be a parent.

There will be times when we have to make a hard or unpopular choice to protect our patients. If we had gone ahead with surgery, there is a good chance that everything would have been OK, but I doubt I would have slept as well as I did that night with my clear conscience.

Trust your gut. In matters of patient care, there is a reason no one suggests erring on the side of recklessness.

3
PATIENT INTERACTIONS

*"They may forget what you said—
but they will never forget how
you made them feel."*

CARL W. BUEHNER

BE KIND TO YOUR PATIENTS

BEING A PATIENT can have its irritations, to say the least. From the inconvenience of getting time off work for the clinic visit, to the long and boring wait before being seen, to the anxiety around one's health and potential treatments, to the apprehension and discomfort associated with the examination. (Full disclosure: when it comes to my *own* eyes, I get queasy!)

So be understanding when you meet with your patients. Try to see things from their perspective. Do everything you can to put them at ease. For those who are old and frail, speak with your staff about booking them when it is more convenient for them and do your best not to make them wait too long.

I once had a patient referred for a two-month history of floaters in one eye. He called our office a week prior to his appointment with questions about his upcoming clinic visit. Specifically, he asked if a three-mirror examination would be done. Typically, for complaints of floaters, I do like to examine the peripheral retina with a three-mirror contact lens. Hence, when the note crossed my desk without providing much detail about the reasons behind the request or the emotional state of the patient, I said yes. The second time he called, he asked if it was absolutely necessary, as he was losing sleep over the thought of the trauma that it would cause him. Understanding the background better, I conveyed that we would not perform the test if he did not consent to it and that we could talk about it when we met.

On my patient intake sheet, I ask, "Do you have any apprehension about the eye examination?" When I see "yes" ticked off, I try to explore what the concerns are and how I can help alleviate or minimize them. A week later, when the patient arrived at the clinic, he checked off "yes," and next to it scrawled "scared about three-mirror examination."

When we sat down and discussed this, the patient described how sensitive his eyes were and the psychological trauma he had suffered after a previous three-mirror examination. He found the thought of repeating it overwhelming. Nervously, he again asked if we had to do it. I did the following:

1. I took the time to explain *why* I would typically perform that examination;
2. I explained what we could do instead and what the consequences would be (without scleral depression or a three-mirror exam, I explained there was a slightly higher chance that I might miss a retinal tear if he had one);
3. Most importantly, I let him make the final decision; and
4. I did not make him feel bad about his decision.

At the end of our encounter, he was extremely appreciative and relieved.

On behalf of all of us with sensitive eyes, here is my plea: if someone is afraid or otherwise challenging to examine, be patient with them. Be careful with what you say and how you react, so you don't make them feel even more embarrassed or bad about it.

THANK YOU FOR YOUR PATIENCE

CLINICS GET DELAYED and patients unfortunately often need to wait beyond their appointment time to be seen by the doctor. Retina clinics can run notoriously behind schedule. By the time patients are registered, seen by the technician, and fully dilated, many are already upset at how long it has taken. In an academic center, prior to the attending popping in, the trip may also include stops with the keen and well-meaning medical student, the tired resident, and the grumpy fellow. It helps to mention the potential for delays when you provide patients with their pre-appointment information. By informing them that they may have to wait, they can appropriately plan their ride, and they'll know to bring medications, snacks, and a sudoku to pass the time.

During my career, I have witnessed various approaches to the issue of the "impatient" patient. There is the option of attempting a joke: "Hey, that's why we call you patients (patience—get it?)!" Some physicians try to explain that delays are inevitable due to emergencies or more complicated pathology. Others try to skirt around the matter completely and dive right into the examination. Whenever he entered the exam room, one physician with whom I worked would always say, "Thank you for your patience. I apologize for your wait." These simple words seemed to placate even the most irritated patients. His patients appreciated that he had at least acknowledged that they were inconvenienced by the wait and that their time was important. Ideally, your practice runs on time. If it doesn't though, this little courtesy will likely restore the patience of that impatient patient.

WEB OF LIES

A LITTLE KNOWLEDGE is a dangerous thing. A little knowledge combined with internet access can be a terrifying thing.

In this age of information, patients are justifiably interested in reading about and gaining insight into their condition and possible treatments. However, the web is fraught with misinformation. Left alone to roam unescorted, unassuming patients can find themselves in the most distressing of places. I find more and more patients are arriving at my office with unwarranted fears regarding their symptoms that were fueled by reading the wrong material on the internet. In our post-truth era, it is challenging for patients to decipher fact from fiction.

You can provide a valuable service by directing patients and their families to good websites. Take the time to find the sites that provide reliable and accurate information on the most common conditions that you treat and that are written for patients (i.e., in simple, non-jargon-laden language).

The best scenario, of course, is to create a website of your own in which you can tailor explanations and instructions to your preferences. This does, however, take a significant amount of effort, time, and money. Your site will be a reflection of your practice and many people's first impression of you, so invest in it well. Ensure it has a professional and polished look, and check it yourself to see that it is complete and does not have dead links or other issues. Also remember that your patients have visual problems (!), so pay particular attention to font size and contrast and other design elements that affect readability.

Be responsible with your wider web presence. As a general rule, make sure that your personal and professional online lives are separated. If you want to engage professionally in social media such as Twitter, Facebook, or Instagram, know that these are much more active endeavors and require a significant time commitment. It becomes very obvious if your feeds are not updated regularly, and this can reflect negatively on your practice. Decide if this is something you personally want to commit to or if you can delegate this function to someone responsible whom you trust to manage it.

Tread carefully, and make sure you and your patients don't become prey on the sticky worldwide web.

WALK A MILE IN YOUR PATIENTS' SHOES

I THINK IT'S a useful exercise to see firsthand what our patients go through and deal with. We can get so busy trying to extract the right information from them or to place them in the correct position that we often forget how nervous or uncomfortable they might be. It is easy to get frustrated with the patient who we feel is not being cooperative. We can easily forget how foreign the experience may be since we are so accustomed to administering it.

Have you ever tried any of the things you ask your patients to do? Have you ever had done to you what you do to them? Try all the AREDS vitamins that you prescribe and see which ones taste bad and which are easy to swallow. Check out the various artificial tears at your local pharmacy and be amazed at how much they cost. Do a visual field test and experience the confusion our patients feel. "Was that a flash that I saw just now? Should I click the button??" Have a colleague do scleral depression on you and you might be more empathetic next time you're pushing around that globe! Have someone perform gonioscopy on you and see if you can sit still, keep your teeth together, and your forehead against the bar!

Ironically, although my craft is healing other people's vision, I have a hard time when it comes to my own eyes. I recall the epic battle of 2001: the first time I tried contact lenses, my stealthy eyelid fluttered like a hummingbird to defend my cornea from the evil contact lens that was being charioted in by the sinister finger of doom. My eyelid fought valiantly and won spectacularly. Sorry, poor optometrist who tried so hard. When I asked a colleague years later to check my angles with gonioscopy, I'll admit I was not much better. It was a reminder of how sensitive our examinations can be.

I'm not asking you to get an intravitreal injection—just make an effort from time to time to see things from your patients' perspective. Sit in their seat and find out how it feels.

KEEP 'EM COMING BACK

YOUR PATIENTS EXPECT good service and they will seek out another physician if they don't get it from you. Poor service complaints often stem from patients feeling that (1) there was a lack of communication from the physician and staff, (2) their questions were not adequately addressed, or (3) there was an excessive wait time to see the doctor.

The first step in trying to improve patient satisfaction in your clinic is understanding how your patients perceive the service that they are being offered. Ask them for anonymous feedback on the clinic. What do they appreciate? What improvements can be made? Armed with this information, you can institute concrete changes to ameliorate the environment and improve patient care.

The qualities patients seek in their doctor include friendliness, approachability, and kindness. In fact, patients often value these kinds of personal attributes significantly more than intelligence or medical knowledge.[9] Patients want to see

---

[9] S. Walsh, B. Arnold, B. Pickwell-Smith, and B. Summers, "What Kind of Doctor Would You Like Me to Be?" *The Clinical Teacher* 13, no. 2 (2016): 98–101.

a physician who listens to them and takes the time to explain things and answer their questions. They want someone with whom they get along, who isn't abrupt, and who doesn't rush them.

Many of us are overworked and have long and busy days. And with stretched resources, we are asked to do more with less. As a consequence, each patient visit risks becoming shorter in duration, with a potential deterioration in the quality of the patient experience. It is a true skill to *efficiently* elicit the appropriate history, politely redirect the patient who is a poor historian, create a diagnostic plan, deliver pertinent information, and appropriately answer any questions—all while ensuring that each patient feels respected. Unfortunately, in order to save time, sometimes we inadvertently end up compromising on the "respect" part. Ideally, methods for increasing efficiencies and saving time in your workday should focus on aspects that can enhance, rather than detract from, the patient-physician interaction. There are fewer legal actions taken against those who take time to talk to their patients,[10] so if for no other reason, spend a few more minutes with them. It is hard to sue someone you like!

It is not uncommon to hear a patient say, "He didn't tell me anything," when describing an encounter with their physician. So either the specialist did not explain things well, or the patient did not hold onto the details. Patients typically do a good job of following what is being said while it is being explained. However, they may not be able to recall the details of the discussion later. I liken this to being driven through an unfamiliar area of town. We all follow the left or right turns as

---

10 B. Huntington, and N. Kuhn, "Communication gaffes: a root cause of malpractice claims," *Baylor University Medical Center Proceedings* 16, no. 2 (2003): 157-161.

they are happening. However, when asked to drive that same route again on our own, many of us would have a tough time.

A colleague and I were discussing this and she told me her approach to this problem. "At the end of the encounter, after I've explained things in detail, I like to review by enumerating the issues. I give the patient a short summary list and I tally it up on my fingers so they can count with me. For example: 'Number one, you've got a cataract in both eyes. We've decided to watch that for now. Number two, you've got dry eyes. We're going to try drops for that, as we talked about. Number three, I want to send you for some tests to check for glaucoma.'"

So there you go—it's as easy as one, two, three!

GREAT EXPECTATIONS

TELL YOUR PATIENT what your intervention will do *and* what it will not do.

When you're caring for people, ensuring that they have realistic expectations is paramount. If the outcome of therapy does not fall within the spectrum of what your patient understood was possible, they are sure to be dissatisfied.

Early in my training, with the guidance of my attending, I performed my first barrier laser for a patient with a retinal tear. At her follow-up visit, everything looked great and the tear was well sealed off. But she was quite upset. "But I still have floaters!" she exclaimed to me in dismay. While *I* was happy that she was stable and had not progressed to a retinal detachment, she regarded the treatment as a failure. This was a good reminder for me that the patient's biggest concern does not necessarily coincide with our main focus. In our discussion with her before her treatment, the attending and I had neglected to elicit her expectations and explain that the laser would not take away her floaters. However, as this was her main symptom, she understood this to be the main goal of the therapy.

Afterward, I sat back and thought about this disconnect. I realized that our concerns and those of the patient varied due to our differential experiences with the issue at hand. I was familiar with the devastating effect that a retinal detachment could have on vision, and I was pleased that we had prevented this from happening. On the other hand, I (thankfully) had never suffered a retinal tear in my own eye and thus had never experienced how annoying (or sometimes debilitating) floaters can be. Our patient had no experience with retinal detachment, so she did not truly appreciate that threat, but she was being driven crazy by her floaters. Had we done a better job of informing her and managing her expectations prior to doing the laser, she still would have had the floaters, but likely she would not have been so upset.

If patients do not expect an outcome, they are more likely to perceive its occurrence as a disappointing and possibly frustrating *complication*. People are distraught or alarmed when they do not get the heads-up. They are more willing to be understanding of negative outcomes or bothersome side effects if we tell them about them ahead of time and they are not a post-treatment surprise. When it's anticipated, a symptom is more acceptable. In general, as long as patients feel that you informed them, were fair, and tried your best, they will be understanding if things don't turn out "perfectly." One patient who'd had the misfortune of requiring multiple operations for recurrent retinal detachments told me later that having realistic expectations markedly helped her from a psychological standpoint. Because we cannot predict how things will go, plan to under-promise and over-deliver.

It is always easier to counsel someone about something that *might* happen than to convince them afterward that it is part and parcel of the process. In our work, it is *not* better to beg for forgiveness than to ask for permission!

GET YOUR HEAD OUT OF THAT SCREEN!

AS I PRESENTED a patient's history and my thoughts on the diagnosis and management plan to my attending, I heard a distracted "umm... hmm" from time to time. When I finished, there was a silence, followed by another "uh huh." "Can you tell me the story again?" he asked, finally looking up from his smartphone.

Our days are full of distractions thanks to those amazing little computers we all carry around. We feel compelled to frequently check our email, respond to our texts, or post on social media. Although our devices help us be more productive and efficient, they can also interfere with polite and respectful interaction with those humans immediately in front of us. We all know the feeling of talking to someone while they are gazing down at their screen rather than into our eyes. And while we know it is rude and do not appreciate it, we are all guilty of it from time to time! Have you ever been to a restaurant and seen a couple who are spending their time on their phones rather than talking to each other? (Are you smiling as you read this because you and your partner *are* this couple?)

I trained with another attending in my residency days who, as soon as he saw you approach him, would put down whatever he was doing, smile, and ask how you were and how he could help. It made such an impression on me. He made me feel that I was important and that he was genuinely interested in hearing what I had to say. Getting someone's undivided attention these days can be a luxury.

Even when we are using a screen for an appropriate purpose, it may get in the way. The increased adoption of electronic medical records has created an abundance of doctors who spend more time looking at their monitor than at their patient. We are at risk of connecting better with medical websites than with those who seek our advice and care. Set an example for polite screen use for the people you train. Be courteous and respectful to patients when you have to use a screen—apologize, explain what you are doing, and when you are able to, listen in a way that shows you are not distracted.

Let's all make an effort to not have screens ruin a perfectly good conversation!

DON'T GET TOO COZY

"THANKS SO MUCH, doc! And remember what I said—you and your wife are welcome to use our cottage whenever you want!"

"That's very generous, thank you," I replied in an appreciative but noncommittal way.

The gratitude that patients have for our work is one of the most satisfying and rewarding aspects of our job. And yet many of our patients want to express their thanks not just with words but also with tangible gifts and offerings. However, this delicate situation can leave us with conflicted emotions. It is rude to not accept a gift; we learn this from a young age. Even when you hate that ugly shirt your aunt gave you for Christmas, you are taught to force a smile and express gratitude. "I love it!" you learned to say through clenched teeth and with a desire to only wear it again on the occasion of your aunt visiting. "The shirt I gave you at Christmas!" she will say when she visits and sees you wearing it. "Oh this? Yes, of course. I wear it all the time!" you will reply in a higher than normal voice that makes you question if the pitch of your response sounds too artificial and gives you away.

With your patients, strike a balance. Don't be rude, but do discourage any gifts that feel over the top. You don't want to drive a wedge in the relationship by having your patient think that you are ungrateful for their gesture, and yet it is not appropriate to accept a gift that is too lavish or large. The latter would threaten the professional physician-patient relationship and your ability to properly care for your patient. You do not want to risk feeling indebted to a patient such that it influences the way that you would approach their care.

There is a reason that our licensing bodies discourage us from treating family members or close friends: our judgment may be clouded due to these close relationships. We may end up being tempted to inappropriately bump them up the waitlist, over-investigate with unnecessary tests or imaging, or make decisions in a different way than we otherwise would have. If you get too cozy with your patients, before you know it you risk moving them from the patient zone to the friend zone.

I was discussing this topic with a colleague who related a story about one of his patients. Every time this patient came to see him, he insisted on offering my colleague tickets to sports events or concerts. Fast-forward a few years and the patient was pushing him to inappropriately "massage" details when filling out long-term disability forms. My colleague reflected, "If I had taken him up on his offers of all those entertainment tickets, I think it would have been harder for me to do the right thing in the end."

The title "Dr." helps to maintain that professional boundary—particularly for those of us who get the "you look too young to be a doctor" line. Occasionally, we get patients who decide to forego formalities and call us by our first name. If ever asked, "What should I call you?" by a patient, a mentor of mine had a great response. Dr. Brian Leonard, former president of Orbis Canada, used to say, "You can call me what my mother called me: Dr. Leonard." He was joking and the patients always had a good laugh about it, but the point was that the relationship is first and foremost a professional one, and there are many good reasons to maintain that.

TRULY INFORMED
DECISIONS

EVERY PATIENT WE meet will have a different motivation for improving their vision and each will also have a different threshold for risk. These differences are influenced by the patient's background, personality, intellect, vocation, attitude toward modern medicine, expectations, and preconceptions, among many other things. Gone are the days of paternalistic medicine when the doctor would make a decision without much discussion with or input from the patient. We must appreciate that what would be best for one person may not work for another. For example, I once had a patient ask me if their epiretinal membrane was cancer. When I said no, they sighed with relief and told me they were happy and did not want surgery. On the other hand, I had an engineer (with better vision than the last patient described) who told me that if there was a chance of making him even 1 percent better, he was ready to sign up!

A good doctor educates the patient and helps them come to the decision that makes sense for that specific patient. A very important part of our informed consent process is helping patients understand what could happen to their condition if they choose not to pursue treatment. In fact, many patients who decide against any intervention are still anxious to know what to expect with watchful waiting. In many instances, the simple reassurance that their ocular condition is unlikely to render them "blackout blind" can have a remarkable effect. This is the deepest fear in the minds of many of our patients, and empowering them with this knowledge can take a huge weight off their shoulders.

I believe it is important to respect the patient's informed decision *and* to support them. It may not be what you or I would do, but we must understand that for *them* it may be the best decision. After I discussed treatment options with a patient for her macular hole, she ultimately chose to forgo any intervention. We talked about it many times at future follow-ups, each time reviewing the risks and benefits and realistic expectations with observation versus treatment. I took the time to understand her reasoning behind foregoing surgery and did my best to address her concerns in a balanced and honest way. In the end, I felt she appreciated the consequences of her decision. I expressed to her, "My job is to explain what to expect with any reasonable treatment options and what could happen if you choose to forgo treatment, and to answer all of your questions. Deciding whether or not to move forward with treatment is your call." When I told her that I supported her decision, she was very grateful and comforted.

In urgent situations, the decision-making process is typically straightforward. For example, very few patients would decide not to move forward with an intervention to repair a globe rupture or retinal detachment. When it is understood that observation will undoubtedly lead to a very poor outcome, almost all patients choose to accept the risks of surgery in the hope of attaining the benefits.

The more challenging situation for patients is deciding whether to move forward with an elective intervention. Many will have difficulty choosing and are ready to do whatever you suggest. It's not uncommon to hear "Whatever you say, doc" (particularly from elderly patients used to paternalistic medicine). The easiest and quickest thing to do would be say, "OK, sure, let's move forward." Fight that urge! With great ability comes great responsibility. Just because we *can* do something, that does not mean that we necessarily *should*. Be careful not to "convince" a patient to undergo a procedure. Take the time to delve again into the risks, benefits, and alternatives and talk to the patient to better understand their motivations for improvement and their acceptance of risk. Never hesitate to bring them back in to discuss things again. That's the nice thing about elective interventions: there is time! Sometimes, the patient needs to review the information on their own so that they can reflect and think of other questions that will help them decide. Many patients are anxious about surgery and can be put more at ease if the conversation occurs over a few visits. It is not a bad idea to check in with them with questions like "Does that sound reasonable?" "Are you happy with that plan?" and "Does that make sense?"

Try organizing your discussion around the following three questions:

1. Is the issue urgent or elective? This will give you the chance to highlight what might happen if the patient decides to forego treatment.
2. Is the treatment in question an accepted and reasonable option? Here you have the opportunity to discuss the legitimacy of the treatment, and the probabilities of associated risks and benefits.

3. Is the patient a reasonable candidate? Not all treatments are appropriate for all patients, and it is important to review this with each patient.

Until you are convinced that the patient is making the right decision for *them*, be cautious about offering to move forward with elective surgery. Unrealistic expectations are hard to meet and may leave you with a dissatisfied patient—even if all goes well from your perspective.

MAKE THE CONNECTION

I'VE GOT FOUR tips for you to help establish a connection with your patients.

I. REMEMBER ONE THING

"How's soccer going?" my family doctor would ask me when I was a kid. I loved soccer—and he would always remember to ask about it.

Years later, during a communications session in medical school, an attending of mine said, "Remember at least one thing about your patient outside of their medical history—a hobby, interest, or recent important event—and write it down in their chart. Ask them about it and it will remind them that they are not just a number in your practice, that you care about them as a person. Even if you are only with them for a short period of time, make it a more human experience."

I really liked the family doctor I had when I was a kid. I realized that a big part of this was that I felt he took interest in me and not just in my illness du jour. (Phantom headaches were quite common, for example, and would start like clockwork a few hours before an oboe lesson; stomach aches were generally used to get out of swim practice; and so on.)

2. WHAT'S IN A NAME?

People appreciate it when you take the time to learn how to pronounce their name properly. Although Shakespeare wrote that "A rose by any other name would smell as sweet," I am sure if the rose could talk, she would tell you just to call her "Rose."

When I am unsure of how to say someone's name, I simply ask them. I have had a few patients say, "No doctor has taken the time to ask me that before!" A trick that someone taught me is to then write it out phonetically in the chart for future reference. Remember that Rose by any other pronunciation would not sound so sweet.

3. KNOW THE ENTOURAGE

Acknowledging the person or people whom the patient has brought with them is the polite and considerate thing to do. However, a word of warning: never assume a relationship. I was pretty good about this. I would always ask the patient, "And who have you brought along with you?" One time, however, I was with a patient who didn't speak much English so I was out of my normal routine. I asked the family member who came along to translate, "And is this your mom?" It just slipped out. "She's my wife," he replied with a frown. Yikes! My face went red as I stumbled through the rest of the encounter. Have the question "Are you family or a friend?" in your back pocket for the patient's entourage and you will not go wrong.

4. LAUGHTER IS THE BEST MEDICINE

People always ask their doctor, "Why did this happen to me?" Often times, the answer in ophthalmology is quite simply old age. Cataract, macular degeneration, glaucoma, dry eye—all these things get worse with age. I thought to myself, *There must be a nicer and more delicate way of putting this.* A few years ago, I started describing this in different words: "As we have more birthdays..." or "As the eye matures..." The patient usually would chuckle and respond, "You mean I'm getting old?" A little laugh can go a long way toward developing a good doctor-patient relationship. In order to help comfort and build trust with patients, think about the subtleties of the language you use and how you articulate your thoughts, all while maintaining a high level of professionalism.

A patient said to me one day, "Never lose your bedside manner. I'm sure lots of people can care for the eye, but not everyone can care for the patient as well."

Keep these four tips in mind to help make the connection with your patients (who are, after all, the reason you chose this profession).

ALWAYS VALIDATE YOUR PATIENT'S EXPERIENCE

I AM ONE OF those people who does not hide their emotions well. If I am bored, my eyes glaze over with ennui and my mouth slacks open as it gives in to gravity. When I am angry, my brow reaches down for my chin while my eyes bulge ferociously. If I were in a silent movie, happiness and sadness would be clear as day to everyone in the audience, whether or not I tried to conceal my emotions.

As physicians, through history taking and physical examination, complemented by laboratory and diagnostic imaging tests, we try to place our patients into specific boxes or diagnoses. In many cases, experienced clinicians are able to clinch the diagnosis just from the history itself. However, we have all had that experience where the patient explains their symptoms in fantastic, vivid detail and it is so foreign to anything that we have come across before that we are not sure in what direction to go. In these moments of confusion, my face wants to scrunch up into a question mark, but I have become (somewhat) adept at hiding at least this emotion out of respect for the patient.

Modern medicine may not be able to explain everything that a patient is describing. We shouldn't forget, however, that the patient is the expert in their own lived experience of the symptoms or illness. If you minimize a patient's story, they may feel that you're not listening to them or don't care. You are missing an opportunity to use the "art of medicine"—connect with them and show empathy. A patient's story and disease are very important and meaningful to them. Everyone has the need to feel validated. So don't dismiss what they are experiencing because it doesn't fit into your understanding of the disease. You don't have to pretend to understand, but at least let them know that you are considering what they've said and trying to figure out how it fits together. Simply acknowledging that you understand that they are experiencing something, but that you cannot necessarily explain *why*, can be empowering for some patients. Remember different people may experience their disease differently. How they describe it may not be what we would expect.

Try it out and you may, from time to time, hear comments like, "You are the first person who actually listened. Everyone else I've seen just made me feel like I was crazy."

CAN YOU SAY THAT AGAIN, BUT THIS TIME SO IT MAKES SENSE?

WE SPEND YEARS learning sophisticated medical terms and phrases, just so we can use them to thoroughly confuse our patients. Even when we try to break down things into more digestible, easy-to-understand language, we sometimes still don't make any sense to them.

"Ma'am, it looks like the jelly of your eye has separated, but I don't see a detachment or tear, so I think everything is fine." Go ahead, admit it. If you are in eye care, you have probably used some variation on these words, at some point, to explain a posterior vitreous detachment to a patient. However, imagine not having the background that you have and read the sentence again. Certainly there is room for clarification! We are probably all guilty of this. From time to time, I have definitely caught myself using language that flies way over my patient's head.

I recall once stopping myself in the middle of an overly convoluted explanation of a patient's pathology. My pause came in response to the puzzled and distressed frown on her face, which was deepening by the second. I realized that while what I was saying made perfect sense to me, I wasn't doing a good job of conveying that information in an easily understandable way for her. I humbly said, "OK, let me start over."

What seems normal and straightforward to us likely will not seem that way to the patient. Although it may be the thousandth time *we* have gone through the explanation, it is probably the first time they've heard it. We sometimes forget this and instead of using language they can understand, we use highly technical medical words and move through what is a familiar script to us. I have seen even experienced clinicians fall into this trap. Being able to provide patients with information in an accessible way does not always come naturally.

I was once seated in the examination room with a patient whose consult had unfortunately gone missing. While my staff members were trying to track it down, I was eliciting my patient's account of why she had been referred to me. She told me that her general ophthalmologist had said she suffered from "sneaky eyes," but that she wasn't able to relay much else from the conversation. I responded with a very intelligible "uh huh" and a blank stare, as I tried to make sense of what she had said. I rarely dismiss confusing statements like this; often it just takes a bit of time to make sense of them. Sure enough, when I examined her eyes with the slit lamp microscope, the patient had posterior synechiae. "Syn-i-chia" or "*sneaky eyes*"?!

The lesson: don't expect our patients to speak our language. It took us years to learn it. In our encounters with patients, we need to speak their language.

THAT MADE SENSE! BUT NOW I DON'T REMEMBER ANY OF IT...

ONE CHALLENGE WE face when providing information to patients is that what works with one person may not work with another. Patients come with varying backgrounds, attention spans, and abilities to absorb new information. Some patients research their symptoms prior to seeing us and arrive with an already strong understanding of their disease. Others are a clean slate when they show up. It is also amazing how stress can compromise our ability to process information. In light of all of this, we must strike that delicate balance—providing enough information to satisfy each unique patient, while doing our best not to drown them with too many details. And with first-time patients, we have to achieve this balance with people who are essentially complete strangers.

I had just finished explaining everything to a new patient who was referred with a retinal detachment. I'd covered diagnosis, pathogenesis, risks and benefits of treatment versus observation, alternatives, and what to realistically expect during surgery and follow-up. "Would you mind if my sister came in to listen to everything you just said?" she asked nervously.

Rookie mistake, Gupta! Rule number one: only start giving information once you've asked the patient if there is anyone in the waiting room whom they want included. (It always surprises me that not all patients think to bring everyone into the room right from the start of the encounter, but this frequently happens.) As I busied myself with filling out the information required by our operating room, I asked *her* to explain to her sister what she understood of our conversation. I was shocked—she did terribly! If this had been an exam, she would have failed. It was eye-opening for me how little information she had comprehended and retained.

I thought back to when I had to take a few weeks off work during my residency due to a left middle lobe pneumonia. My visit with my respirologist was the most impressive encounter that I have ever had as a patient. Not only did he explain everything very clearly, but he gave me written educational information to reinforce what we had discussed. Although I worked in healthcare, I did find the material very helpful, as I realized that I would not have otherwise been able to recall all that we had talked about. At the conclusion of our interaction, he "checked in" with me: "Does all that make sense?"

In a time when more and more patients are taking an active role and interest in their health, it is good to be able to send them home with a summary or review in some form. Create your own written handouts. Shoot some videos for your office's website. Read online patient materials so you can direct your patients to the reliable sites.

Take the time to not only explain things clearly but also to check in to make sure that your patient has understood everything and then take steps to make sure that they will retain the information as well.

NOTE I actually suffered a left lower lobe pneumonia. The left lung does not have a middle lobe. (Just making sure you are awake!)

I GOTTA FEELING

"THEY MAY FORGET what you *said*—but they will never forget how you made them *feel*." Dr. Brian Leonard, a mentor of mine from my residency days, would often remind us of this quote from Carl W. Buehner. And although Buehner was not talking about patients, he may as well have been. In fact, studies show that patients immediately forget about half of what their physicians say to them.[11] And of the material that they recall, significant portions are typically incorrect. Of course, given the potential stress of the encounter and the unfamiliar subject matter, this is not surprising. Your tone and demeanor when interacting with your patients are just as important as (or perhaps even more important than) the words you articulate. Consider the cadence, clarity, and calmness of your speech as you connect with patients. Even if you think you are saying reasonable things, if your tone is dismissive, your patient may leave with a bad experience.

I can recall a patient interaction that seemed to be going well from my perspective. Mr. W. had been referred to me for

---

[11] R. Kessels, "Patients' Memory for Medical Information," *Journal of the Royal Society of Medicine* 96, no. 5 (2003): 219-222.

what appeared to be either exudative macular degeneration or central serous retinopathy. After I explained my thoughts on his condition and my suggested management plan, I noticed that he seemed to freeze up. It quickly became obvious to me that he was getting overwhelmed. I paused as I carefully considered my next words. I chose to address my sense of his emotions head-on. "You seem upset. Can you tell me what you are thinking?" Unfortunately, he'd had enough and wanted to conclude our meeting and make an exit. Before he left, I very quickly but calmly conveyed to him that I could meet with him again at any point to go over things once more if he wanted. I also expressed that I would be happy to refer him to another specialist if he preferred that option. I told him that I understood how changes in one's health can be upsetting and that I was here to support him and offer him whichever option he felt most comfortable with.

Several weeks later, Mr. W. returned to see me. What came out of our conversation was exactly what Buehner was referring to: Mr. W. did not remember much of the content of our conversation, but he felt good about his visit. He told me that he'd felt respected and able to trust me, and had wanted to come back and revisit our discussion when he was ready.

Dr. Dean Cestari, a neuro-ophthalmologist at the Massachusetts Eye and Ear Infirmary, put it nicely when he said, "If you haven't made the patient feel better than they did when they walked in the door, you haven't done your job."

TOUGH QUESTION!

WHETHER YOU LIKE it or not, difficult patient questions and scenarios are guaranteed to arise at some point or another. Just as you prepared for the tough scenarios that you know you will almost certainly see on your examinations, get yourself ready to handle the tough patient questions. There are great advantages to planning what you might say in advance. Don't leave it until the critical moments when they pop up; your emotional reaction in the heat of the moment will likely be less than satisfying for both you *and* the patient. Have a strategy in place for how you would ideally like to reply. Visualize yourself getting these questions and sensing emotions from the patient and responding to them. Think of helpful language and phrases that you can employ. Practice with friends or family.

Let's look at a scenario together. Your patient is *extremely* nervous when you first meet him. The fear of the unknown can be very unsettling and anxiety provoking. It has him very tense and almost ready to burst with worry. "Everything will be OK, right? It's not serious, is it?"

In these situations, it is not uncommon for *us* to *feel* the patient's anxiety. Their anxiety becomes *our* anxiety. Our natural response is to want to resolve the emotional distress. We want to be able to tell them, "*Yes!* Everything will be OK. It's probably nothing!" and watch a wave of relief wash over them. Unfortunately, we can't often make that immediate promise. One thing that can prove helpful is to first *acknowledge* your sense of their feelings with a statement and then to *ask* what is at the root of their concern. For example, "You seem anxious. Am I correct? Is there something specific you are worried about that we can discuss?"

Our job is to be honest with the patient but to do so with empathy and embrace the human side of healing. A calm response is helpful, conveying that while we cannot guarantee any specific outcome, we will give our very best care. At times, I express that while I wish I could tell them that everything will be OK, we have to take things one step at a time. It can be reassuring for the patient if you clearly list next steps regarding imaging, blood tests, referrals, etc., to show there is a plan in place.

I have found that knowing and reflecting on my instinctive emotional response in this type of scenario is very helpful. Whereas before I felt unable to control the apprehension I would experience, I now force myself to decelerate my speech. I deliberately focus on my breathing and my heart rate and try to slow them. I pause before I talk so I do not interrupt the patient, and I ensure that they have finished expressing their thought completely. When I force my body to be calm, my mind follows suit, allowing me to do my best to help comfort the patient.

To review, in the scenario of the *extremely* anxious patient, I have found the following five points helpful.

1. Avoid the temptation to resolve emotional distress by making baseless assurances or being too definitive about a prognosis.

2. Acknowledge their emotions and ask about the root of their fears.
3. Convey that while you cannot guarantee an outcome, you can guarantee your best efforts, care, and support toward the best outcome possible. Temper hope with realism.
4. Focus on maintaining a calm demeanor.
5. Reassure them with next steps: "Let's take things one step at a time."

Here are a few other challenging questions and comments that you may encounter at some point. I encourage you to think through how you would respond.

"How am I supposed to work like this?"
"I'm so scared of surgery!"
"Am I going to go blind?"
"What would you say if I were your mother?"
"I've been waiting too long to be seen! This is ridiculous!"
"You look so young! Have you done this before?"
"Shouldn't my last doctor have seen this or picked this up?"

Whenever I am faced with delivering difficult news or feel that my patient's expectations will not be met, I think of the words of my friend and colleague Dr. Adrian Fung: "Not everyone can be cured, but everyone can be cared for."

BETTER THAN THE BOSS

WHEN YOU ARE in training—whether during residency or fellowship—always remember that you've got to be better than the boss. Most patients will automatically be hesitant to have you perform a procedure on them (or even examine them) due to your trainee status. And to make things worse, to many patients, your youthful looks scream *"lack of experience!"*

One of the challenges of learning the craft of ophthalmology is that many of our tests can be somewhat uncomfortable for the patient. And the longer the exam goes on, the more unsettled the patient may become and the harder it may be to extract the information you require. (Contrast this with radiology or pathology, where images or slides will wait around all day and remain cooperative until residents can figure out what they are seeing.)

So what can you offer the patient to gain their trust? The first step is understanding what most patients look for in an interaction with a physician: they want to feel respected, they want to be heard, and they don't want to be rushed. And for any procedure, they want to feel as little pain and discomfort as possible.

Spend more time with the patient than your attending would be able to. Anesthetize them well, and explain things fully and clearly. For anxious patients, elicit their specific concerns and fears related to a procedure or exam, and address them. Turn down the lights you are shining into their eyes to the lowest intensity you require to appreciate the fine details. Develop a deft touch in all your exams. For example, when placing a gonioscopy lens or posterior pole lens on the eye, strive to use the minimum amount of force necessary.

There is nothing more disconcerting to a patient than seeing their doctor fumbling around with equipment or seeming unsure about how a machine works. If you don't inspire confidence, the patient may not give you a chance, even if, in the end, you would have done a good job. Not only will you have lost a learning opportunity, but future trainees may also lose out as a result.

So, as you work toward the day when you actually *do* know what you're doing, at least *look* like you know what you're doing!

WHAT'S THE (FULL) STORY, MORNING GLORY?

THIS WAS MY second visit with Mr. A., a middle-aged gentleman with visual decline due to a relatively dense cataract. Unfortunately, his fellow eye had not seen well since birth. During our first encounter, I got the sense that he was very resistant to the idea of surgery. At the same time, however, he was clearly conflicted, as his vision loss was now significantly impacting his daily life. I described the details of the surgery, its risks and benefits, and what he could realistically expect from the intervention if he decided to move forward with it. We agreed to meet again in a few months so he could think things over.

At our second encounter, Mr. A. was no readier to make a decision and was clearly struggling. Finally, I asked the question that I should have asked earlier: "What is holding you back?" "My aunt lost an eye after she had a cataract operation," he replied. That was the critical piece of background information that I had been missing. And it is quite possible that if I hadn't asked Mr. A, it would have stayed buried. So I delved further into the details. His aunt's surgery was done in the old days of extracapsular cataract extraction. From the sounds of things, she developed a severe infection in the eye.

Sadly it could not be saved and was removed in the end. I was able to explain to Mr. A. that while the small risk of an infection with surgery was unavoidable, modern-day incisions were much smaller and the surgery quicker than in days past. Just having the conversation—even though I could not give him a guarantee—gave him some relief. Until then, all his anxiety had been bottled up. Now that it was out in the open, his fears could be addressed in an honest and frank way.

People may be resistant to sharing information for any number of reasons. Most often it is because they are either embarrassed or scared. We need to identify the barriers that cause our patients to not adhere to or participate in a treatment plan. In some cases, their reasoning will make complete sense. But in others, their reasoning may be misguided and an easy solution may be present. What's holding them back? Is it cost? Fear of pain? Time off work? It is not about convincing them but about dispelling myths and giving an honest evaluation and assessment to allow them to come to an informed decision.

When in doubt, simply ask your patients directly if they are worried or scared about the examination or procedure. That starts the conversation. Ask them if they know anyone who has already had the procedure. If they do, they may come with all sorts of preconceptions about it. Sometimes a patient thinks that because it didn't work on their neighbor, it won't work on them. Or since their cousin got it done and everything went well, it should be a guaranteed success.

We have a challenging job. In a limited number of interactions and focused amount of time, we have to tease out our patients' misconceptions, fears, concerns, and biases and address them in an honest and forthright manner. We only typically get a snapshot of who our patients are. We see whatever they choose to present to us during the doctor-patient interaction in the very one-dimensional setting of our office. We do not see the full fabric that is their life. Only by asking can we gather useful and important information that the patient might not share otherwise.

We can inform patients all we want, but if we don't get their side of the story and understand what baggage they are coming in with, we may miss the opportunity to help them.

YOU CAN CHOOSE YOUR FRIENDS, BUT YOU CAN'T CHOOSE YOUR PATIENTS

MY FELLOWSHIP MENTOR and I had just spent forty minutes discussing retinal detachment surgery with a patient with a very challenging personality. Once the patient had left the room, my mentor looked at me and said, "You can choose your friends, but you can't choose your patients." Simply put, no matter a person's personality or personality disorder, that patient still deserves your best effort.

Throughout your career, you will encounter thousands of different people. While it can be fun and interesting to interact with the broad variety of personalities and backgrounds that comprise the human spectrum, you will have to take the good with the bad. We need to expect that some of our patients are going to be more anxious, nervous, scared, argumentative, belligerent, fickle, smug, vindictive, sensitive, impatient, and emotional than we would like.

One subset of patients will withhold information. They may believe that if you do not ask specifically about something, it can't be the cause of their problems. Or they may be testing you to see if you meet their expectations. Whatever the reason they are doing this (and unfortunately for them), you may be led down the wrong path and pulled away from the correct diagnosis.

These are the personalities that are analogous to the tough clinical or surgical cases. Anyone can get a great result in the easy surgical case or clinch the diagnosis in the simple, straightforward medical presentation. In the same way that we should strive to get the great outcome in the complex surgical cases and make the correct diagnosis in the confusing clinical presentation and rare diseases, we should make it our goal to excel with the five-percenters with a difficult personality. These patients will not always agree with you. They may not always be reasonable with you. Recognize that even a minor disagreement with one of these patients on any aspect of their medical care or surgical outcome can lead to a major problem if not properly addressed. Even if the medical care you provided was appropriate, if they do not see it that way, some may go out of their way to make things difficult for you.

Understanding and accepting that difficult patients will come into our offices will, hopefully, allow us to have better interactions with them, keep our cool, and help them feel respected, comforted, and well cared for. The challenge is that these patients have a tendency to bring out the worst in us. Be prepared—they do not come in wearing a sign! You have to be on alert to identify them in a crowd so that you can try to prevent their personality from affecting the true goal of the interaction, which is to preserve or enhance their health.

YOU CAN'T WIN 'EM ALL

THE SPECTRUM OF humanity includes every intelligence level, personality eccentricity, opinion of physicians, political leaning, religious conviction, and slant of possible discrimination. We will occasionally meet patients who think we are too young or too old, too dark or too light skinned, or too whatever. These people may not be able to leave their ageism, racism, sexism, or any other –ism at the door. They bring it along with them when they come to see us and it can color their interaction with us.

I had an odd experience with this. My administrative assistant left a message on my desk saying, "Mrs. W. wanted to let you know that you misdiagnosed her. She would like you to call her back to discuss this with you." *Interesting*, I thought. Mrs. W. had commented on my boyish appearance when we met. Perhaps that was at issue here. I remember spending a significant amount of time explaining to her the cause of her problem, as well as the risks and benefits of observation versus the various reasonable treatment options. As her vision still measured quite well, I had asked her to return in a few months to discuss everything again before moving forward with any intervention. She had not returned.

"Young man," she said when I phoned her back, "I got a second opinion and wanted to let you know that you were wrong." Mrs. W. then went on to describe to me (with several inaccuracies in terminology) her correct diagnosis. I calmly asked Mrs. W. if it would be OK if I read back to her the dictation I'd sent to her referring doctor. In the letter, I had described my conversation with Mrs. W. at our visit and concluded with the same diagnosis that she had just relayed to me (minus the imprecisions).

I mulled over this strange experience. Where had I gone wrong during my initial visit with Mrs. W.? In the end, I wondered if this encounter simply fell into the category of "You can't win 'em all." I could not help but feel that no matter what information I conveyed to Mrs. W. or how I approached it, she may not have heard me. She seemed to be focused on my youth, which she may have seen as inexperience.

In most interactions, your goals and those of the patient will line up. Invariably, however, you will encounter patients who will not be on the same page as you. From time to time, you will have to deal with someone who has a different agenda. We need to always keep in mind that what seems reasonable or appropriate to us may seem unreasonable to them, due to their background or the opinions they bring to the interaction. This discordance can lead to nonadherence to treatment, unproductive and inefficient investments of time and energy on your part, and complaints. These scenarios will bring you mental stress and cause you to lose sleep. Your challenge is to identify these patients as quickly as possible, so that you can do your best to minimize the harm they may create for themselves and for you.

WORST BEHAVIOR

SOMETIMES, WE ARE on our worst behavior when it is most critical that we be on our best. In the heat of an emotional exchange, our judgment becomes clouded and all we want to do is win the fight. We lose sight of the actual crux of the discussion and fall into the "win by any means necessary" mentality. We yell, we say things we do not mean, we walk away or offer the silent treatment. Given the right circumstances, it does not take much for most of us to allow the five-year-old inside of us to dictate our conduct.

Know that this is normal and that it is going to happen. Accept it. Like anything else in life, it takes practice to improve our behavior. In fact, try losing an argument! Get some humility. Everybody likes to be right. So if it isn't a big deal, let it go. Allowing someone else to be right and to "win" an argument can sometimes be more powerful than digging in your heels and fighting to be right yourself. Remember if you find yourself burning all your bridges, you risk ending up alone on an island on fire with no way off.

I have always loved the saying, "I will listen to you, especially when we disagree." Use this with colleagues, family, friends, and total strangers alike.

Patients can come to you with some pretty far-fetched ideas. If their position is not going to harm them, don't spend time unnecessarily trying to discount a belief that is deeply entrenched. If you are not going to be able to convince them otherwise and there is no risk of harm to them, let them be right. Remember your goal is to preserve or improve the patient's health. To do so, you need to be able to work together. A patient with strong convictions who does not feel you respect their perspective will be less likely to adhere to any plan you try to put into place.

A patient was sent to me with decreased vision secondary to exudative macular degeneration. He was convinced it was due to dust getting in his eye the week before. I explained that we would not normally connect that sort of event with the change we were seeing in his retina and explained the typical risk factors for the disease. I could tell he was still committed to the dust theory. "In medicine, I never say 'never,' and I never say 'always,'" I offered. Rather than fighting him by focusing on what we would not agree upon, I tried to work with him and shift our focus to our common goal, which was to stabilize his vision. This he could get behind.

Know that difficult patients are bound to come your way at some point. Mentally prepare for them so that you are able to stay on your best behavior. If you have a patient in your practice who is known to be challenging, plan ahead. Book them for the last appointment in the day so you can give them the time and attention that they will demand. Play out the interaction in your mind while staying calm as you think about it. Mentally play out common scenarios. Consider the patient who gets upset with the wait time and aggressively accosts you or your team members. What will you say or do to de-escalate the situation? Imagine the anxious patient who emotionally asks one pointed question after another. How will you calm them? Think about the unhappy postoperative patient who objectively has a good outcome but who is miserable. How will you validate this patient's symptoms while addressing his misperceptions?

We also often have to tell people things they don't want to hear about their health. People respond differently to this sort of information with reactions that can include anxiety, anger, mistrust, spite, disappointment, frustration, bitterness, and fear. Unfortunately, these emotions may be misdirected against us—even though we are trying to help. We'd love to tell them, "Don't shoot the messenger, shoot the disease! We're on the same team." Our role is to stay calm and help the patient through the range of emotions they'll experience on their road to healing.

The patients whom you dread seeing are probably the ones with whom you should spend more time. Don't let them draw you in and upset you. Show them that you are listening to what they have to say and that you care. Some people are scared, some are upset, and some are just unreasonable. Take a deep breath. Listen. Stay calm. Be empathetic. Be accommodating. Be patient. Don't let your inner Incredible Hulk come out.

4

LIFE LESSONS

"A goal without a plan is a wish."
ANTOINE DE SAINT-EXUPÉRY

"A GOAL WITHOUT A PLAN IS A WISH"

I LOVE THIS QUOTE. It is attributed to the French writer Antoine de Saint-Exupéry, although I'll admit that I was never a big fan of his. I only read *Le Petit Prince* because I was forced to in grade school. In fact, I only came across his words of wisdom in a sports documentary analyzing why professional athletes go broke. Herm Edwards, then coach of the New York Jets, addressed an audience of young football players in his typical animated and larger-than-life style. He quoted the French author to emphasize that we do not achieve things in life by simply leaving them to fate.

We all have things that we would like to do—improve our physical fitness, learn a new language, pick up a new skill, or take an idea to market—but so many of our ideas and intentions fail to transform themselves from wishes to tangible accomplishments. Why is this? When things are busy and we get into the cycle of the everyday grind and only see as far as the end of the day or week or even month, we don't allow ourselves to work on long-term goals. Those, however, are the ones that really allow us to grow and make a difference in this world.

My friend Adrian Salamunovic, cofounder of the very successful company DNA 11, once gave me some amazing advice. He is a guy who is overflowing with enthusiasm and a love of life. Adrian asked me to list my five-year goals. I brainstormed on multiple ideas I had always wanted to pursue if I ever had the time. As I was speaking out loud, I realized I was describing wishes rather than goals. Sure enough, Adrian's next question to me was "What is your plan to get there?" That night, I went home and I committed my goals to paper. There is something about writing it down—either in pen or electronically—that helps me get things done.

When creating a timeline for your plan, ensure it is a realistic one. Revisit it on a regular basis—every six months, for example—to see how you are coming along. Give yourself enough time to actually make progress so you do not become discouraged and give up.

Find a mentor and make use of their advice and guidance to help you understand what you want to do with your career. If patient care is your only focus, that's great. My hope is that, whatever you choose, you come to your decision after having thought through all other avenues—research, medical education, teaching, advocacy for the profession, policy work, administration, speaking at meetings, involving yourself in societies, or advocating for approval of new medications, instruments, and surgical interventions.

When you look back on your career, what do you want to have accomplished? Do not regret leaving these as wishes—make goals now!

MAKE YOUR SLOPE A LITTLE STEEPER

NOT MUCH SEPARATES one little kid from another. For example, I'm certain that my curriculum vitae at age four would not have been far off Elon Musk's at that age. I could pick out my colors and rhyme off my shapes with the best of them. With subsequent years, however, the CEO of Tesla and SpaceX has shown himself to be one of the most innovative minds of our time. On the other hand, I still routinely confuse my dark blue socks with my black ones.

While few of us will ever attain the success of the Elon Musks of the world, we can at the very least strive to be a better version of ourselves.

When I was thirteen years old, all winter I pushed my cardio training to the max, in the hopes of being selected for the all-star soccer team come spring tryouts. Every time I finished my workout, my mom asked, "Did you give it 110 percent?" As a moody know-it-all teenager, I would reply that her question did not make mathematical sense and that one could only realistically give a maximum of 100 percent. My mom would just smile in response.

My mom was trying to drive home an important lesson. That additional 10-percent push can be the difference between getting the job or not, between securing the grant or losing out, and between making the soccer team or fantasizing from the sidelines. Indeed, the more important thing to realize is that the extra effort, in the end, pays dividends many times over. Each time you succeed, you are provided with more opportunities to grow and achieve. Those who make the soccer team get more elite coaching and mentoring. They join skilled teammates in practicing more challenging drills. They get exposed to tougher opponents, elevating their level of play and strategy. As the saying goes, "The rich get richer."

Over the years, I have sat on many different admissions committees. I have been amazed by the caliber, diversity, and experience of the candidates. And I have been even more amazed by how little separates those who make it from those who don't.

The world is a competitive place! So what gives you a leg up on the next candidate? Be aware that large unproductive gaps in your CV may stand out unfavorably in the eyes of a selection committee. Take advice from the London Tube and its warning: mind the gap!

Imagine your life trajectory as a slope on a graph. Dig a little deeper, push a little harder, and make your slope a little steeper!

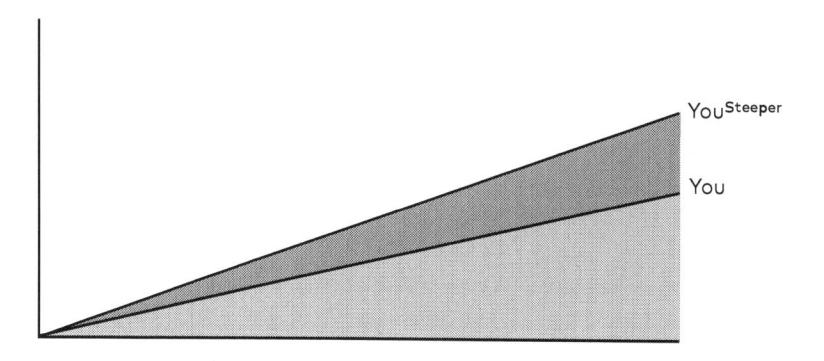

WHAT'S YOUR GREATEST STRENGTH?

IT WAS THAT time of year again: interviews were taking place to select the new group of residents. My fellowship supervisor, Dr. Michael Kapusta, and I were in the OR idly discussing classic interview questions.

"What would your answer be if I asked you to name your greatest strength?" I asked him.

"That's easy," he replied. "My greatest strength is that I *know* my strengths and weaknesses *really* well." I frowned as I processed this. Was this a brilliant and insightful response, or was I being trolled? Before I could decide, he continued, "And my next greatest strength is that I know the strengths and weaknesses of those *around* me really well." Before I could get him to expand on that, our attention shifted to the surgery at hand.

A few years later, I was participating in a wonderful workshop called Engaging Others. One of the faculty was making the argument that it is important for us to understand not only our own strengths and weaknesses but also those of the people around us. My mind was taken back to Dr. Kapusta's response to my question. Brilliant and insightful, I reluctantly concluded.

During the course, we were asked to fill out a questionnaire that was created by the consulting company Gallup.

Their strengths-based leadership assessment would highlight our top five strengths and categorize them into the domains of (1) executing, (2) influencing, (3) relationship building, and (4) strategic thinking. When I received my personalized report, I saw that my top five strengths were distributed between domains 2 to 4. The column under the heading *executing* was empty, however. This came as a surprise. Surely I was good at executing. Wasn't I? And yet when I showed these results to anyone else—family, friends, mentors—no one was shocked. "You are chronically taking on new ideas and projects and never finishing any of them!" was the common theme. In a quote often attributed to Friedrich Nietzsche, he said that "sometimes people don't want to hear the truth because they don't want their illusions destroyed." Smart man. So, there I was, wallowing in thoughts of the unfinished manuscript from medical school, the music album that was in progress for years, the shelved business idea to start a watch company that I was so passionate about... The list went on and on. Yes, the truth is sometimes a cold shower.

So I found out that I am really good at idea generation, team building, and formulating strategy but really crummy at executing and pushing past the finish line. The good news is that once we develop a good sense of (and actually accept) our strengths and weaknesses, we can start intelligently building a team with the appropriate strengths to complement us where we falter. To do this, we have to understand the strengths and weaknesses of others.

While it took me three years and a two-day course to figure out what Dr. Kapusta meant in the OR on that fateful day, I finally got it. Better late than never, they say.

If you can't name your strengths, congrats—we have at least now established one of your weaknesses!

IF WE WERE ALL THE SAME, IT'D BE A BORING WORLD

PHINEAS GAGE.
Does that name ring a bell? If not, you have been missing out! Now I don't want to build the story up too much, but it is one of the most fascinating and remarkable cases in the history of all of medicine. (I didn't build it up too much, did I?)

Phineas was a foreman many years ago on a railroad construction site, just outside Cavendish, Vermont.[12] Part of the project required blasting rock to clear the path for the rails. Holes were drilled in the rock, and then it was Phineas's job to place explosive powder and a fuse inside these holes and then to pack it in with a tamping iron. This crowbar-like tool measured about three and a half feet and weighed more than thirteen pounds. At 4:30 p.m. on Wednesday, September 13, 1848, Mr. Gage suffered an incredible accident that would forever put him in the history books. You guessed it—while performing his duties, an explosion occurred, propelling Phineas's tamping iron into his cheek, up through

---

12 M. Macmillan, "Restoring Phineas Gage: A 150th Retrospective," *Journal of the History of the Neurosciences* 9, no. 1 (2000): 46–66.

his frontal lobe, and out through his skull. It landed thirty yards away.

Remarkably, Mr. Gage was able to ride unsupported on an oxcart back to his residence, where he would be examined and treated by a Dr. John Harlow. Although Phineas would recover physically over the subsequent months, psychologically he was a changed man. Harlow reported a radical alteration in Phineas's character—describing him as impatient, irreverent, fitful, and grossly profane. Now, if I'm being honest, I think if a metal rod ripped through my skull, I might become a bit more impatient too. You can just imagine a clueless friend of Phineas saying, "Hey man, what's gotten into you lately?"

They say that you can choose your friends, but you can't choose your family. And for many of us, the same holds true for our work colleagues—we can't choose them either! Post-injury Phineas was an extreme example of someone who might have been difficult to work with. When we understand *why* Phineas behaved the way he did, however, we probably have more empathy for the way he handled himself.

While it must have been hard to miss that Phineas Gage was dealing with some serious stuff (hole in the head), many people's troubles are concealed from those around them. We never really know what people are dealing with. Keep this in mind, and try to give people the benefit of the doubt.

The fact of the matter is that we are not necessarily going to get along with every person we come across. Nor will we agree upon all issues that come up. And that's OK! In fact, some of the best ideas are conceived as a result of differences

---

NOTE In 2002, I crossed off one item from my medical bucket list: I saw Phineas Gage's *actual* skull and tamping iron! If you are ever in Boston, take the time to go the Harvard Medical School's Warren Anatomical Museum and you too will get to see this remarkable exhibit!

of opinion and *respectful* debates. Respectful debating means that the dialogue centers on the *issues* and finding common goals, rather than criticizing and attacking perceived character differences.

The next time you have a challenging time with *that* person at work, take a deep breath and let it roll off you. Be the bigger person—don't give into temptation and allow the relationship to spiral out of control. You don't have to be best friends but, for the common goal of the patient, figure out a way to maintain a healthy professional relationship. Ask yourself, *Will this matter in ten years?* Try to identify and focus on their positive attributes. Work on not allowing your coworkers' actions or words to affect your feelings; that is giving them too much power and control over you. Be the master of your own emotions. It is a very liberating feeling!

Throughout your life, may you meet the full rainbow of backgrounds, personalities, attitudes, aptitudes, and approaches that the world has to offer. Respect and embrace others for who they are—*especially* if they are different. This helps us grow and makes us stronger. If we were all the same, it'd be a boring world!

SOMETIMES THE SQUEAKY WHEEL GETS THE GREASE, AND SOMETIMES IT GETS REPLACED

"**Y**OU KNOW WHAT the problem is?"

We waited for this week's rant. By now, we were all accustomed to every meeting opening with the same person vocalizing his concerns. One member of the committee rolled her eyes and two others sighed and slumped in their chairs. Unfortunately, each week, it was becoming more and more difficult to focus on the actual content of this person's comments. Rather, all we heard was his whining and complaining tone. Even when he made good points, they carried less weight because we had half tuned out. Many of you have probably participated in meetings just like this.

They say that the squeaky wheel gets the grease. Yes, it is true: no one can help you effect change unless they know there is an issue. If you bury your head in the sand and quietly suffer, people might just assume that things are hunky dory. But nobody likes a complainer! If a wheel gets *too* squeaky, rather than getting greased, it might just get replaced.

So pick your battles—not every issue should be a crisis. Learn when to push for things and when to let them go. In the heat of the moment, we usually have a lot to say, and our clouded judgment tells us that others will receive this "valuable" information and be brought around to our perspective. This, of course, is rarely the case. Realistically, there are certain things that you may just have to endure. Part of your decision-making about what you can and can't live with will relate to the dynamics of the relationship and the nature of the issue.

You have probably heard the advice to "write the email but not send it." Over the years, this has saved me many times from creating an awkward or uncomfortable situation for myself. When I reread those emails the next day, they get heavily edited or, often, deleted.

Even the specific words we employ can have a powerful influence on the people around us. Can you feel the difference between "You know what the problem is?" and "I think one of the bigger challenges we need to consider is…"? The former feels more forceful, while the latter welcomes others to contribute. For some listeners, the word *problem* may have a more negative connotation than *challenge*. Reflect on the language and phrasing you use, as well as the tone of voice you employ, and consider the percentage of time you spend speaking versus listening. When raising your concerns, choose the right approach for a given audience, and you'll likely be met with less eye-rolling and more support.

I have a policy of "Don't just bring the problem; bring the solution as well." Often the person who has recognized an issue is best poised to solve it. Those who need to be involved at a higher level in the decision-making may not have even realized that there was a problem—let alone thought through how to fix it. If you take initiative and invest the time to explore the options, there is a better chance that the solution chosen at the end of the day will be the one that also works best for you!

Put things in perspective and decide which issues are worth fighting for. Remember you only have a certain amount of "complaining" currency to borrow from people. After a certain point, they may stop lending an ear and you may end up bankrupt.

GO WHERE YOU WANT TO BE

WHERE DO YOU want to be when you set down your roots? In your heart of hearts, what place would you most like to call home? Pick the country, state, province, or city, and say it out loud. Maybe this place is important to you because of family. Perhaps you love it because of the mountains and the skiing. Is it your passion for the big-city buzz and excitement that draws you? Or are you attracted by the affordability of a smaller community and your ability to buy a big house for your kids to run around in? The place might represent a unique research opportunity that you can't turn down. Or maybe your reason for liking it is as simple as the weather.

Whatever your decision, there will be trade-offs, as every opportunity has its advantages and disadvantages. Particularly in your first job, it's rare to have it all. For most positions you consider, you'll be the low person in the hierarchy.

Often the choice drills down to either taking less money and being where you want to be or making more and being farther away from the things you are passionate about and the people you love. So forget the money! Take the long-term perspective. Yes, those early years may be leaner, but if you do good work, your practice will build and you will advance in your career.

Like Dorothy said, "There's no place like home." If you're not where you want home to be, promise yourself you'll work to get there soon.

PLEASE, TELL ME
HOW YOU *REALLY* FEEL

"AT TIMES, YOU are too timid in the operating room. You need to be able to react quicker and you need to get more efficient. And for the love of God, if I have to tell you one more time to..."

I'll spare you the last part of the discourse (or more accurately, I'll save myself the embarrassment). Unfortunately, these comments from my fellowship supervisor carried much truth and seared like a fresh wound. I managed to stifle a "please, tell me how you really feel." But I *had* sought out this feedback on my own accord. Suddenly, in my mind's eye, I saw myself as Tom Cruise in *A Few Good Men*, demanding the truth, and Jack Nicholson roaring back, *"You can't handle the truth!"* This incident occurred early in my fellowship and I wanted to know what I could be doing to improve. How did I compare to previous fellows? Where did my perceived weaknesses lie? What could I do to be the best fellow they had ever had? They say don't ask for honest feedback if you can't stomach the response! While my immediate sentiment during this interaction was one of unease, soon after I was glad I had sought out this information, as I knew in the end it would make me better and be worth the pain.

A bruised ego presents an incredible opportunity to learn and to improve. The challenge for all of us is to be humble and open to the (hopefully constructive) criticism and to not get defensive. Too often, our subconscious immediately and automatically seeks out justifications for what we did or how we behaved and rationalizes why we should not change. It is a natural instinct to protect one's self, one's reputation, and one's pride, but in these instances, we need to suppress this urge to be defensive and to fight back. Process the information in an analytical way and set aside the emotions that may blind you to real and fixable issues. Isn't it better to know and have a chance to change than to live in ignorance missing an opportunity to improve? Don't allow yourself to resent the person critiquing you. Thank them! Even if you feel they are truly off base, there is likely some fraction of truth to what they are saying. Seize on that opportunity to develop.

While *hearing* honest feedback can be hard, it can actually often be challenging to *give* an honest evaluation. Most people don't want to hurt other people's feelings or to create confrontation or discomfort in a relationship. For some evaluators, the path of least resistance is to say that everything is OK, rather than to take the time to do a proper and detailed assessment. Unfortunately, this approach does a major disservice to the learner. And unless you, as the learner, recognize that this is happening and make an effort to extract this important information, you will miss an opportunity to improve.

Think of your favorite mentor. What is it about this person that allows you to listen to and accept constructive criticism from them? Now think of a person with whom you do not see eye to eye. What is it about your interactions with them that gets your back up? Is it possible that both might be conveying the same information to you, but you're only accepting it from one of them? Remember that everyone has something to offer and teach you. However, since they may not be the best at articulating it, it will sometimes be up to you to figure out how best to draw it out of them. As you progress in your career from student to teacher/mentor, you too should work on how to deliver negative or constructive feedback that is timely, valuable, and impactful.

There are times when you may suffer from evaluation overload. In some programs, trainees are evaluated daily. Then there are 360 evaluations, where everyone evaluates everyone. Quantity does not always mean quality, however, and there is a risk of feedback fatigue for both evaluators and trainees. Learn to look for the common themes that come out of all this feedback and focus on those.

Remember, as a physician, you have committed yourself to lifelong learning to increase your knowledge and enhance your skills. Accepting feedback and making changes accordingly are inherent parts of this journey. So embrace the evaluations (good and bad), just as you embrace new evidence and technologies, and watch yourself grow as physician, teacher, and person.

TIME FLIES (MAKE SURE YOU'RE ON BOARD)

AS THE LAST of my things were loaded onto the moving truck, my mom smiled and said, "The days were long, but the years were short." I laughed. A rush of memories came back to me as I realized how right she was. It had been an amazing two years of fellowship training, packed with ups and downs. I saw myself mature as a surgeon and grow as a person. The days were certainly busy, however. I remembered when my folks visited one Christmas when I was on call, and they barely saw me due to the onslaught of urgent cases. While many individual days felt long at the time and ended late, the years did somehow zip by.

Remember how the fun days of summer seemed to last forever when we were kids? And now, with every blink, it feels like a season has changed? There is the old saying that time flies when you're having fun. Well, an equally appropriate saying would be that time accelerates as you grow older. If you are nodding your head as you read this, you are not alone experiencing this. This concept has been reported in the psychology literature, and it is indeed a common phenomenon for people to perceive time passing more quickly as they age.

So a few more years disappeared and before I knew it, I was married and settling into a new job and a new city. To my bewilderment, my wife and I were having weekly meetings with lawyers, accountants, and financial planners; there was estate planning, organizing for retirement, drafting of wills, arranging disability insurance, and deciding on life insurance.

It's the beginning of the end, I couldn't help but think to myself. Just as we were finally ready to *start* life in one sense, we were drowning in paperwork to ensure it *ended* well. It was enough to tip me into a midlife crisis. What did I want in life? Would I have the time to accomplish it? Or was life just going to pass me by, one routine week at a time? I spun out of control worrying about the future and poring over the past.

One day, while I was still in this funk, I met Mr. K., an incredibly engaging and remarkably youthful ninety-two-year-old patient. (One of the things I love most about the field of ophthalmology is that we get to interact with the elderly. It fascinates me to meet people in their nineties and hundreds—what have they experienced in triple my lifetime?) Mr. K. loved sports. He explained to me that he had to stop skiing ten years earlier. I was amazed—he was skiing at the age of eighty-two?! He asked me if I golfed. I replied that it was something that I always wanted to do but never had found the time to learn. I admitted to him that I thought perhaps it was too late in life for me to start. "I started golfing quite late," Mr. K. countered.

"When did you start?" I asked.

"When I was eighty," Mr. K. replied.

"Huh. I guess it's not too late for me to start then." I chuckled as I calculated the forty-five-year head start I would have on him.

We have the opportunity to learn so much about life from our patients and their support people. Over the years, I have learned about courage, resiliency, strength, gratitude, empathy, acceptance, patience, hard work, and dedication. Mr. K. taught me that while life does pass by quickly, it is never too late to make a change or start something new. There is no time like the present! Before he left that day, he drove the point home: "Live in the present. Too many people have their head stuck in the past or are worrying about the future. Enjoy the moment and relish the experience at hand and the people with whom you are sharing it. You never know when you are going to get it again."

Treat time as your most precious commodity and live purposefully and mindfully in the moment to ensure the weeks and years do not slip through your fingers. In one of my favorite comic strips, *Calvin and Hobbes*, wise little Calvin remarks, "Know what's weird? Day by day nothing seems to change. But pretty soon, everything is different."

IF HE CAN DO IT, I CAN TOO!

NOT ALL AREAS of medicine were created equal. In my humble (and *extremely* biased) opinion, ophthalmology is definitely the coolest. However, it is also (again, in my view) one of the more challenging ones to learn. It is neat to reflect on the variety of skills that we learn during our training, most of which demand exceptional hand-eye coordination. To excel, we require a very delicate and nuanced touch and a sophisticated appreciation of subtle alterations in the anatomy of the most beautiful organ in the body. From the different lasers to the assortment of minor and major procedures, there is definitely a lot to learn and then master. Even in our clinics, we make use of so many instruments that it's almost like being in surgery but without the incisions!

I clearly remember feeling overwhelmed in my first year of residency while trying to improve my skills in slit lamp microscopy, retinoscopy, gonioscopy, and scleral depression, among many others. *Am I ever going to be good at this?* I asked myself the question that every one of us has uttered at some point. And every time that thought would creep into my head, I would quiet it down by remembering a story that a family friend had told me when I was little. Writing exams stressed him out, until he learned a little trick. When he would start to feel overwhelmed, he would sit back in his chair and look around the room. Invariably, he would see someone else in much worse shape, scratching their head and looking even more frantic. "If he can do it, I can too," he would say. This would calm his mind and give him the confidence to push forward and succeed.

Since first hearing this story when I was a kid, I have regularly used it to get my mind out of "woe is me" mode and into "yes I can!" mode. I remind myself, *Well, if they can do it, I can too!*

When I went scuba diving for the first time, something about the tank and the mask made me feel claustrophobic under the water. While we were learning to breathe with the tank in shallow water, I started to feel extremely uncomfortable and felt my mind spiraling out of control. I abruptly stood up out of the water, thinking, *Oh no! I'm not sure I can do this! Am I going to be left on the boat to talk to myself while everyone else explores the beauty of the ocean?!* I stopped myself, took a deep breath, and, in my mind, revisited a conversation with a friend who had learned to dive the year before. I told myself, *Darn it, if Kathryn can do it, I can too! Get under the water!* That one little saying kept me from missing out on the fun.

We sometimes have to guard against imposter syndrome. We may feel like we've just "made the cut" or that we've fooled everyone and we're simply imposters among others who are *truly* deserving. Don't think that you're the only person who has found something difficult. If you struggled with something on the board exam, it's safe to say that others did too. In all likelihood, if something is not clear for you, there are others in the room confused about the concept as well. To reach residency or fellowship, you have had to be pretty successful in life, work hard, and be reasonably intelligent.

Be confident in yourself and your abilities and in your capability to improve and learn and succeed!

ALWAYS LOOK LIKE A WINNER

DURING OUR TRAINING years, or even as junior attendings, many of us look quite young. This may play on the minds of our patients, especially the elderly. Subconsciously, many of them worry that our youthful features signify a lack of experience. They'll nervously ask, "Are you old enough to do this?" or say, "My, you look so young! Have you done this before?" This is their way of expressing anxiety about you treating them. Be prepared for questions like this. No matter how you plan to answer, take extra time with these patients, thoroughly answering all their questions and making a human connection to gain their confidence and trust and to put them more at ease. Dressing unprofessionally or looking sloppy will not help your cause. I was given good advice before my first day of medical school: "Dress well—you've got to at least *look* like you know what you are doing!"

It is challenging to care for a patient who does not have confidence in you. And nothing deflates the air of a patient's metaphorical balloon of confidence more than watching their doctor fumble around and look confused. You can, of course, fumble around and look confused on your own—just not in front of your patient! Supplies go missing. Technology fails.

The last person to use the machine may have altered the settings. Sometimes you might forget which switch is which. These things happen to the best of us, and they do not necessarily represent our expertise and ability. That being said, sort it all out first and *then* bring the patient in the room.

One day, a resident working with me came out of the laser room more quickly than I had anticipated. "Problem?" I asked. "Not sure how to turn on the laser," he replied. At my look of surprise, he explained that all of his previous laser experience was with a different model. He was not familiar with this system and had simply assumed he would be able to figure it out. Of course, while he fiddled unsuccessfully with various buttons, the patient watched with increasing alarm and dismay. How *Not* to Inspire Confidence 101. I joined my resident in the room and ran through the laser interface's nuances. If he had taken the time to review things and set them up *before* bringing in the patient, he would have been fine. Not doing so led to the patient questioning his competence and losing confidence. It's not that he wasn't competent; he just wasn't organized. (I recall doing pretty much the exact same thing when I performed my first pneumatic retinopexy. Like I said, it can happen to the best of us!)

There are days during residency, fellowship, and independent practice that can be tiring—emotionally, mentally, and physically. Be organized. Sit up straight. Dress professionally. Speak clearly. Stay cool under pressure. Convey confidence. Fight through it to be positive, energetic, and pleasant, even when you're down. People around you will appreciate your attitude. Even when you're under stress, try to not let the nurses, patients, or rest of the team feel it. They will see your emotions and reactions and respond in turn. Stay calm and work through the issues. Always look like a winner!

LEARN TO SAY NO

JIM WAS AN overachiever who always said yes when offered an opportunity or asked for a favor. You could always count on him.

Does this story sound familiar? Could we easily substitute "Jim" for your name?

I am going to tell you something groundbreaking and liberating. Brace yourself. Are you ready?

You do not have to say yes to everything.

I repeat: you do not have to say yes to everything.

David Allen, the author of *Getting Things Done: The Art of Stress-free Productivity*, reminds us that we "can do *anything*, but not *everything*."[13]

Of course, we all *know* that we *can* say no. So why is it hard for us to do so? Well, for starters, we often feel like we would be disappointing the person who's asking. We feel obliged to say yes and guilty about saying otherwise. At times, this is complicated by a power differential, which may cause us to contemplate potential secondary consequences of saying no.

---

13 David Allen, *Getting Things Done: The Art of Stress-free Productivity* (New York: Penguin Books, 2001).

Or we may worry that if we say no, there will be no one else available or qualified enough to take our place. Finally, being the go-getters we are, it is always tough for us to live with our own FOMO (fear of missing out).

One trick to avoid becoming overcommitted is to step back before saying yes to something. Ask if you can look at your schedule and think it over and get back to the person later with an answer. This will give you time to reflect. It will separate you from the moment and the immediate feeling of obligation. Keep in mind that you will not be doing anyone any favors if you cannot do a good job because you have taken on too much or are not really that interested in or committed to the project. Be mindful not to spread yourself too thin. Be fair to yourself as well as to those depending on you and expecting you to deliver.

Ask yourself what your priorities are at this stage in your life. There are, of course, some things that you *have* to do. Include these in your considerations, then list and rank the rest and commit them to paper. Understand that priorities may change with time. There will be things that are important to you but that can wait for when other immediate priorities are not in your direct path. In five years, perhaps you could participate in something that you do not have time for now. Do not fall off the treadmill of ambition because you set the incline and pace too high.

They say shoot for the moon and if you miss, you'll land among the stars. While that sounds romantic, let's take a second to remind ourselves what a star is: a burning ball of gas. Our sun, for example, is a star. As you might expect, landing on a star would be a horrible fate. There are some very compelling reasons why you have not heard NASA discussing a mission to land on the sun—the first of which is that the sun's core is believed to measure fifteen million degrees Celsius. So, while I still do like this saying, I read it more as a cautionary tale. I would say that if you are not prepared to properly shoot for the moon and you end up missing and landing on a star, you'll burn out. So be aware of your limits.

THESE ARE MY CONFESSIONS

MY WIFE HAPPENS to also be an ophthalmologist. As a result, we've always seen eye to eye. (*Pause for laughter.*) Yes, dinnertime conversation is often eye opening. (*Pause for laughter.*) All right, I'll stop—sorry! She had just gotten off the phone with a colleague who graduated around the same time as she did, and she relayed the conversation to me. While the dialogue had drifted over a number of topics, most of their discussion had centered on the challenges of starting independent practice. They had commiserated over tough cases and traded stories.

Especially early in our careers, it is nice to have someone whom we can bounce ideas off, review cases with, and get advice from. For some of us, this probably happens organically. If that's not the case for you, consider seeking guidance and counsel from colleagues in your department or from your previous teachers. Mix it up—conversations with mentors who are at a later stage in their career may offer you something different than, but just as valuable as, chats with contemporaries. As well, the more formal morbidity and mortality rounds in your department can be complemented with more informal chats over coffee.

We all want to do our best for the patient and, in every case, we hope that our best is good enough. However, when things do not go as expected, showing vulnerability and being able to discuss complications and mistakes requires strength. It is not healthy to bottle these things up. Your patients need you to be mentally and emotionally well! In fact, it can be very therapeutic and cathartic to be able to talk about medical and surgical errors. Why? Here are some of the reasons why this kind of conversation is valuable:

1. It serves as a reminder that none of us is infallible.
2. It fosters a culture of honesty and transparency, engendering public trust in the medical profession.
3. It is educational and allows for the sharing of strategies others have used to minimize errors in similar situations, and it may lead to finding innovative new approaches to avoid recurrence.
4. It allows for an understanding of the extent and frequency of errors, permitting a systems-based approach to identifying root causes of the problem and to implementing collective efforts toward minimizing recurrence.
5. For the physician involved, it serves as a sort of "confession"—a way to unload their burden and talk about feelings of guilt, sadness, frustration, shame, disappointment, anger, regret, remorse, and shock, among other emotions.
6. For those listening, it offers an opportunity to support, reassure, validate, comfort, and remind those who have erred that they are not alone.

So, since we've set the stage, I will share a less-than-brilliant moment from my medical school days. (You're smiling already,

I'm sure.) I was on my obstetrics and gynecology rotation. My attending stepped out the room, leaving me with a simple enough task: provide the patient with an injection of contraceptive medication in her arm. *Sure, no problem*, I said to myself coolly. I picked up the syringe firmly and carefully directed the needle toward the young lady's deltoid. The needle depressed her skin and I started my injection. Fluid dribbled down the patient's arm. We both watched her contraceptive pool on the examining table. Awkward pause. "I'll go get Dr. P.," I offered quietly. Yes, confidence and competence are two very different things. Unfortunately, I had neither. After cleaning up my mess (literally), my attending patted me on the back and threw out some comforting words, "There's lots to learn, but you'll get it."

As a friend once told me, "Medicine and surgery require resiliency to not be crushed by the defeats and to retain the thirst to grow, adapt, and improve in response to the setbacks and stumbles." Strive for success and keep the conversation going!

I DID EVERYTHING I COULD

WE ALL COME across very complicated and difficult cases from time to time. Some patients have very bad disease. Others seem to have very bad luck. Worse still are those patients who are dealt a bad hand and then play it very poorly. (Think of the patient with labile diabetes who chooses not to regularly monitor their sugars.)

Most patients who experience a bad outcome will still greatly appreciate your efforts if they feel you genuinely did your best for them. During my fellowship training, we were referred a patient with postoperative cataract surgery endophthalmitis. The bug was very virulent and after a less-than-robust response with intravitreal injections of antibiotics, we brought the patient to the operating room for a vitrectomy late at night. In the end, unfortunately, she still had an extremely poor outcome. What will always stay with me, however, is the gratitude that she had for our efforts. Even in light of the fact that we were not able to save her vision, she was so thankful that we had done everything that we could to help her.

When the disease starts winning the battle, your patient will need, more than ever, to hear that you care about them.

They will need to know that you empathize with them and wish they didn't have to go through this; that you know they are disappointed, and you are disappointed too; that you understand this is difficult for them; and that you'll do everything you can to help them get through it.

Throughout our careers, we will encounter patients whose health will unfortunately go downhill, no matter what we try to do for them. However, our goal with each patient is to formulate a good plan so we can honestly say, "I did everything I could," as opposed to "I wish I had done…" If you strive for this, you will be able to take some comfort in the fact that even if a case does not go well, you would not have done anything differently.

DON'T FORGET!

WE ARE ALL human and we all forget things. This is never truer than when our attention is being split by multiple disruptions and responsibilities. Additionally, during our training and early years as an attending, we are at a higher risk of being pulled off track by an interruption than we are later in our careers when much of what we do feels automatic.

To reduce those "oops, I forgot" moments, it is important to employ strategies that work for you. For some reason, during fellowship, I would sometimes forget to create an inferior peripheral iridotomy (PI) intraoperatively in patients getting a silicone oil tamponade. Finally, I made a mnemonic for myself. I started referring to silicone oil as "silicone p-oil." The simple addition of the "p" helped remind me of the need for the PI.

As another example, it was not uncommon while I was operating, for one of the nurses to pass on a message for me from the clinic. Because I was focusing on the surgery, the message would sometimes slip my mind. To help myself, I simply asked the nurses to leave a note in the area where I keep my charts.

When you are doing something new or something that you do not regularly do, it is even more challenging to remember everything. It is, therefore, critical to know how to quickly and reliably access information you might need. For example, if you are a general ophthalmologist in a remote area, from time to time you may have to do a vitreous tap and inject for a postoperative endophthalmitis. While you may not have the drug dosages memorized for the antibiotics or be comfortable with the exact steps and considerations when doing the tap and injection, you should be prepared to quickly access this information. Having the information in a notes file on your phone may be the best approach, but also keep a written back-up in the clinic. If you have forgotten something more than once, it's time to figure out a system to prevent it from happening again!

Being prepared is key to staying out (or getting out) of trouble.

DON'T LET THE FALL CRUSH YOU

DURING OUR LIFELONG pursuit of bettering ourselves in our craft, there are peaks and there are valleys. Never does this ring truer than during our training or first year of independent practice.

Sometimes the valleys can feel really deep... really dark... and really lonely.

After a particularly tough case that I took to heart, a mentor of mine saw that I was struggling. "Don't let the fall crush you," he said. "Your heart and head were in the right place. There are a lot of people who will need you. Don't let single setbacks stop you from growing so you can help all those others who will need you."

Medicine has come a long way, yet there are still many diseases and conditions for which we lack the technology or understanding to be able to heal our patients. In some cases, people present too late; in other cases, they present with something too complex for the tools we have at hand. There will be problems that we won't be able to fix. There will be eyes that we cannot save. Although that does not sit well with any of us, we have to be able to accept that reality. For some physicians, this is more difficult than it is for others.

We all take pride in our work and it is not easy for us to live through failure.

It is normal to feel grief when an outcome is not what we would hope for. I love this evocative quote from the French vascular surgical pioneer René Leriche: "Every surgeon carries within himself a small cemetery, where from time to time he goes to pray—a place of bitterness and regret, where he must look for an explanation of his failures."[14]

Finding the time to grieve is important. Feel it. Be upset. Be angry. Be sad. Be frustrated. But then control and contain it. Break down the case with a colleague or mentor and take time to reflect.

During an OR day, we may need to compartmentalize and delay this emotional process and be ready to pick ourselves back up quickly in order to give our best for our next patient. Resiliency is an extremely important quality to develop. We owe it to our patients to be strong.

Keep these two sayings in your back pocket for the inevitable rainy day:

1. When nothing is going right, go left!
2. Whenever I feel blue, I remind myself to start breathing again.

---

[14] René Leriche, *La Philosophie de la Chirurgie* (Paris: Flammarion, 1951). Translation attributed to Roberta Hurwitz.

AN ERROR IS WASTED IF YOU DON'T LEARN FROM IT

DESPITE OUR BEST intentions, things will sometimes not progress as ideally as we would have wished. Although every error is an unwanted outcome, it is also an opportunity to learn and grow. The period of time immediately following an error is a critical branching point. Are you going to be the person who internalizes the incident and reflects on it in order to improve your ability? Or will you be the type who shakes it off and forgets about it? The next time you are faced with the same scenario, will you end up with the same negative results?

Make it your goal to learn from your setbacks, so that you never make the same mistake twice. If you do not, the chance to improve and do better for your patients is wasted. Carve out time to reflect. Ask yourself, *Why did this happen? What could I have done to have prevented it? After the error occurred, how did I handle the error? Did I do what I could to minimize its negative impact? Could I have done something better?*

Minimizing errors sometimes only requires simple, but intelligent, changes to the way you approach things. For example, when verifying if you have the correct patient, saying

"Please tell me your name" is a much better approach than "Are you Ms. ___?" If the patient is hard of hearing or mishears what you said, it's easy for them just to say yes. Sometimes people are so sick and tired of sitting in your waiting room that they might take any opportunity to be seen next. Now you are potentially set up for disaster if you proceed with the wrong chart and don't realize it.

Create an error log and be disciplined about using it. This strategy will force you to think more about your errors. In addition, it will deny you the opportunity to completely forget about the episodes or to diminish their importance or frequency. During my two years of fellowship, I created a file of errors that I had committed. Anytime I did something that wasn't ideal or optimal, no matter how small the miscalculation—issues with everything from draping to anesthetizing the eye, peeling membranes, repairing retinal detachments, or placing secondary intraocular lenses—I wrote it all down. I would regularly review this list, particularly the night before an OR day. My goal was to ensure that I did not repeat any of the errors I had committed in the past.

When I began writing this chapter, I dug up my error log and had a look through it. During my first few scleral buckle cases, it seems that I had a few in which I split one of the rectus muscles when isolating them with the silk ties. Several weeks after the first incident, I documented that I did it again. There was obviously something that I needed to change in my technique. I can recall discussing this with my attending and breaking down ways of decreasing the likelihood of this happening again. Flipping through the log, I see that I did not commit that error again during my fellowship.

Be vigilant and work hard to improve your techniques and minimize errors. As my fellowship director, Dr. Michael

Kapusta, said to me during my training, "As soon as you get too casual or careless, you'll have an office full of mistakes." When errors do occur, be honest and forthcoming about them, not just with yourself but also with your attendings and your patients. Honesty and humility will go a long way toward building and maintaining the long-term trust that will help your colleagues and patients see beyond isolated mistakes.

NO REGRETS

WHEN I WAS a kid, I was a big fan of the show *Sliders*. (I put this chapter near the end of the book just in case you are familiar with the show and are now appalled at my taste in TV.) In each episode, Jerry O'Connell leads a group of ill-fated travelers through a wormhole into a parallel Earth. They are continuously "sliding" from one reality to the next, always trying to find their way back to Earth prime— their original parallel. The series fascinated me and made me dream about possible parallel realities to my own. I fantasized about being able to play out each life branch on the tree of outcomes that stem from any one decision.

Picture the infinite number of possibilities that you have pushed into oblivion simply by choosing to be exactly who you are today. There is a lifetime of experiences lost as a result of any decision. Imagine being able to go back and experience all the lives of the alternate you's. What would you do first?

Decisions confront us on a daily basis. Most are small and inconsequential. However, from time to time, we are faced with choices that will have a significant impact on our trajectory through this existence. Sometimes the best option seems obvious. At other times, things are not so clear, and this is when we agonize over what to do. These are the times we wish we could "slide" from one reality to the other to see which turns out better.

In the absence of your own wormhole to a parallel Earth, do your best to live out each experience in your mind. Close your eyes and imagine each of the scenarios as vividly as possible. What are the benefits of selecting one route? What are the potential downsides? Consider all parameters and go through the exercise of making a grid to be able to logically compare the choices. Do all you can to determine which of the choices you believe will be best for you.

When you finally make the decision, know *why* you are making it. Identify the rationale behind what you are planning to do, and be sure that the benefits outweigh the negatives. Really internalize why you are choosing this path. Be comfortable with this decision. And, more importantly, know what you are going to question about the decision later. This will prepare you to quiet the voice that may one day whisper in your ear, *Was it the right choice? Would I have been happier if I had decided the other way?*

While the travelers on *Sliders* (stay with me) were continuously trying to get to home, take comfort in the fact that you are home already. Enjoy it. We are going to work with the presumption that you have access to only one world. Don't get lost in thoughts of wishing you were in another one. There are probably a lot of worse parallel Earths out there.

So once a decision is made, move on and close that door. Don't revisit parallel realities again and again. Stay here in Earth prime and have no regrets. Move forward and be happy.

HOW DO YOU DEAL WITH DEFEAT?

WHEN I WAS very young, while playing outside at our summer cottage, I fell down a well. I hit the bottom painfully and there were bats flying all around me. I was terrified. After I was rescued, someone close to me said, "Why do we fall?" I wiped a tear as he answered for me, "So we can learn to pick ourselves back up again." Or wait... maybe that was a scene from the movie *Batman Begins*. Either way, moving on...

We are all used to success. To get to where you are now, you have worked determinedly and sacrificed a lot. More often than not, you have achieved what you set out to do—and everybody loves getting what they want! But what do you do when things don't go your way? It is bound to happen at some time or another. Perhaps you will not get the fellowship you envisioned. It may be that the job you wanted does not come through. There is no doubt that there will be a period of time when disappointment and frustration are appropriate and acceptable. Thereafter, however, are you able to control your thoughts and emotions and separate yourself from negative energy? How will you behave? Will you be bitter? Petty? Will you carry the setback with you and wear it on your sleeve? Or will you rise above it, accept it, and be at peace?

Don't be defined by your defeats. When presented with an unfavorable situation, determine if there is anything practical and reasonable that you can do to alter the outcome. If there is, go ahead and do it. If not, accept the outcome and be at peace with it. I promise you will live a more liberated and stress-free life!

When I finished my surgical retina fellowship training, there was no job available in the country. I kept positive. I recall one of my attendings being amazed by how calm I was, given the situation. I explained that worrying would not help my cause. Instead, I kept knocking on doors and looking for opportunities. Happily, things did eventually work out but not before I got the opportunity to sit with failure for a long time.

As Judi Dench's character, Evelyn, says in the film *The Best Exotic Marigold Hotel*, "The only failure in life is the failure to try. And the measure of success is how we cope with disappointment."

DON'T LIVE IN RELATIVE POVERTY

I GREW UP in a small city where 99 percent of the people were fair-skinned. My brown complexion made me feel like a superhero in the summertime—I never burned! Meanwhile, most of my friends looked like lobsters after a long day of playing soccer in the sun. They would commiserate with each other over the discomfort that would ensue from the blisters and peeling and wince when someone (me) would purposefully slap them on the back or belly.

Not burning wasn't even the best part for me. There was sex appeal to dark skin! When the other sex started noticing me, there I was with a built-in tan. To get my bronze, I didn't have to go to the beach, cook in a tanning salon over the winter, or waste my dimes on a spray-on orange glow. I was au naturel. Ads and media routinely sent us the message that tanned skin equated a life of fun, success, and affluence. Being in the sun was a good thing.

Then, on one of my earlier trips to India, I made a fascinating and startling discovery: everyone there was yearning for lighter skin. Staying out of the sun was a top priority. Skin-whitening creams with offensive ads and brand names like Fair and Lovely were staples in powder rooms all over the country. Girls were told that if they were too dark, they would be hard to "marry off."

As a kid, I did not really have many "grass is greener" moments. Everything is taken care of for you when you're young, and my allowance and toy collection were not dramatically different from those of my more well-off peers. I think this is why I can so vividly recall the moment when I made the absurd discovery that people at opposite ends of the world were thirsting for each other's shade of skin and going to great lengths to achieve it.

Humans are all alike: we want what we do not have. No matter how much wealth, love, and success a person has, there is always someone who has more. We all know that person who works less and makes more money and whose life seems charmed. Focusing on these disparities can lead to jealousy and self-pity. Life is short, so don't spend it worrying about what others have that you don't. Be thankful for what you have and don't live in relative poverty.

ATTEND YOUR OWN FUNERAL

WHAT DOES EVERY person who was born in 1859 have in common?

Give up?

My apologies for being so morbid, but they're all dead. And unless you're reading this book from a futuristic time in which the secrets of immortality have been unlocked, it's a guarantee that at some point you are going to join them.

So here is the scenario: you are dead.

Yes, I want you to imagine that the time has come, that you have crossed over, so to speak. Picture yourself standing at the back of the room as people filter into your funeral. (I would ask you to close your eyes, but then you would not be able to read any further.) Whose faces do you see? Are your family and friends present? Do you see work colleagues, sports teammates, fellow orchestra members, or brothers and sisters of faith? Do you see people with whom you have lost touch?

What would all these people say about you? What qualities, if mentioned, would make you smile as you watched from the back of the room? How would you like to be remembered? Are there specific things that you would like to have achieved?

Are any friends missing from this scene, because distance and time have caused you to drift apart over the years?

This dark exercise is a way to force you to consider how you have been prioritizing the people, activities, and endeavors in your life that are important to you. There are very few people who, on their deathbed, wish that they had spent more of their hours working. And one truth in this world is that none of us knows what the next day holds; unlike milk, we do not come with a known expiration date to help with the planning.

Time flies when you are busy (whether you're having fun or not). Invest now in the people attending your imaginary funeral. Do so with your time, attention, and love. Whatever accomplishments you would like included in your eulogy, make these a priority now. Do not wait until your *actual* funeral; live your life how you would want to be remembered.

I had a patient who used to always tell me on his way out the door: "Hey doc, you know you shouldn't take life too seriously... 'cause you'll never get out alive!"

REFLECTIONS OF A PUPIL

I LOVE MY JOB. Yes, there are days that are longer than I'd wish and more complicated than I'd choose. However, when I ask myself if I am happy with my choice of profession, the answer is a resounding yes.

Most of us *are* happy early in our careers. So how do we keep that feeling? How do we prevent ourselves from slipping down the path of the jaded? Maybe it is by remembering how we got here. What did we say in our medical school interview when we were asked why we wanted to become physicians? To help people—wasn't that it?

My grandfather passed away the year I was born. He struggled with diabetes for many years and eventually lost his eyesight to the disease. When my mom told me this, I was young and I can remember my first thought being that if I couldn't see, I wouldn't be able to play my Nintendo. It was the first time I imagined a world without sight. And it scared me.

Most of us—me included—take our eyesight for granted. We gaze at the world without always appreciating how miraculous it is to *see*. It is a privilege to care for people in their time of disease and disability. Knowing that my work helps people maintain what my grandfather lost keeps me grounded. I like to think he would be proud.

For the hard times, when the system has you irritated, perturbed, and discouraged, remember what brought *you* here initially. And then buckle up for the ride—it promises to be an amazing one.

ACKNOWLEDGMENTS

I HAVE BEEN LUCKY to have had so many distinguished teachers and colleagues over my medical and ophthalmology training, and I am grateful to have benefited from their collective wisdom. I wish to particularly thank the following for their mentorship, support, guidance, and friendship: Dr. Ike Ahmed, Dr. Danah Al-Breiki, Dr. David Almeida, Dr. Kashif Baig, Dr. Rama Behki, Dr. Catherine Birt, Dr. Jason Blair, Dr. William Britton, Dr. Ralf Buhrmann, Dr. Michael Butler, Dr. John Chen, Dr. Netan Choudhry, Dr. Alan Cruess, Dr. Donald D'Amico, Dr. Karim Damji, Dr. Gilles Desroches, Dr. John Dickinson, Dr. Michael Dollin, Dr. Adrian Fung, Dr. John Galic, Dr. Steven Gilberg, Dr. Julius Gomolin, Dr. Bernard Hurley, Dr. Michael Kapusta, Dr. Vladimir Kozousek, Dr. Wai-Ching Lam, Dr. Brian Leonard, Dr. Michael Myles, Dr. Marcelo Nicolela, Dr. Daniel O'Brien, Dr. Michael O'Connor, Dr. Vivek Patel, Dr. Karim Punja, Dr. Flavio Rezende, Dr. Arif Samad, Dr. Shaun Singer, Dr. Sweta Tarigopula, Dr. Raman Tuli, Dr. Devesh Varma, and Dr. Setareh Ziai.

I am extremely grateful to my amazing editor, Cynthia Lank, for her tireless energy, wonderful ideas, positive spirit, and for her ability to corral my thoughts without losing my message. This book would not have been possible without her. Thanks to Donald Sedgwick for his wisdom and guidance in helping me navigate the world of publishing. Thank you to Trena White and her tremendous team at Page Two for their help in bringing this book to life.

Thanks to Mom and Dad, Mom and Pop, Shikhar, Didi, Ashwin, and Shreya for always being there.

Thank you to my patients for the privilege of caring for your precious gift of sight.

Finally, words cannot express my appreciation for my wife, Anuradha, and her patience, love, and encouragement and for always making me smile.

ABOUT THE AUTHOR

DR. GUPTA grew up in St. John's, Newfoundland, where the weather is so rugged that you can't help but have a good sense of humor. After studying biochemistry at Memorial University of Newfoundland, he completed medical school at the University of Toronto. Thereafter, he slowly moved back out east, with stops in Ottawa for residency training in ophthalmology and Montreal for a vitreoretinal fellowship. He was thrilled to settle in Halifax, Nova Scotia, back on the ocean, and surrounded by East Coast hospitality. Dr. Gupta actively participates in research and has published articles in several prominent peer-reviewed journals. He regularly teaches medical students and residents about the exciting field of ophthalmology. He has received awards for his work in medical education, research, teaching, as well as excellence in patient care. Dr. Gupta has a keen interest in preventing physician burnout, achieving a good work-life balance, and strategies to improve overall patient satisfaction. He was instrumental in the creation of a mentorship program for junior Canadian retina attendings. Outside of work, he enjoys sports (playing and watching), music (playing and listening), and hanging out and making funny faces with his son, Vikram.

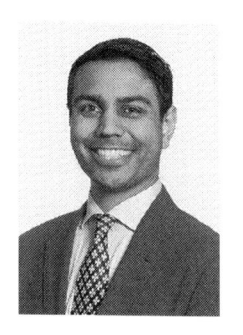

Printed in Great Britain
by Amazon